Reboot:

A Novel of Bipolar Disorder

Reboot

A Novel of Bipolar Disorder

By

Jane Thompson

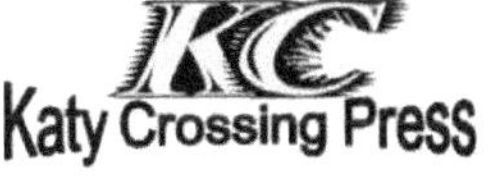

Roboot: A Novel of Bipolar Disorder

By Jane Thompson

Published by Katy Crossing Press, LLC
Georgetown, TX
http://www.katycrossingpress.com

ISBN-13: 978-1477661567
ISBN-10: 1477661565

Cover art: Ross Carnes

Photographer: Ralf Kittenbacher, Artisan Photographix

Chapter One

The old, grey battered metal desk acted as a barrier between Marie and her client.

Marie, looking harassed, was trying to fix the unfixable again and in record time, of course. The black woman in front of her, black and blue and swollen around her face, had three little ones in tow.

Unenthusiastically, the lady asked, "Can you get my husband out of jail by tomorrow? We want him home for Thanksgiving."

"What was he arrested for?"

'"Domestic violence."

"Yes, I can see that."

The beige phone shrilled.

Marie rolled her eyes. At the bottom of the police department totem pole, she had no one to screen her calls. The woman sat stolidly.

"Hello."

Marie was startled to hear Ted's voice on the line. He never called her at work and she hadn't heard from him in three weeks. Her voice lightened and her heart jumped. Then she asked, "hey, what do you want?'

"Well, I hadn't heard from you in a while and I just wondered if you wanted to get a cup of coffee. I should be downtown in the next couple of days."

He never, in the four years they had been seeing each other, asked her for any kind of a public date. He was always afraid that someone would see them and it would get back to his wife. She didn't blame him for that, but it seemed portentous that he was suddenly asking her to go out. She was a bit puzzled.

Marie smiled reassuringly at her client, whose kids were unnaturally, obediently standing still and being quiet.

"Of course, that would be fun. I would be happy to."

Okay, I'll see you then."

"Bye."

She turned back to her client, a huge smile on her face.

"I'll do my best to get your husband out of jail. Just sit here for a few minutes and I'll be back."

Marie fairly flew to the elevator of the jail, knowing underneath the giddy happiness that she had sold herself out. The last time Ted left her apartment after their date, he said, offhandedly, "You know I only went out with you because I was drunk."

She didn't answer, mainly because she couldn't think of one. She didn't go back to their meeting place, the little bar in downtown Oklahoma City that served newsmen and lawyers and was known to all not by its real name but as the "Bar" bar because of the large pink neon sign that spelled out "BAR" over the front door. That was the first time in their four-year relationship she had avoided him In fact, she had purposely tried not to put herself in his path. She had always managed to be where he could easily find her so he didn't have to go out of his way to pick her up. When she stopped going to the Bar, she thought she would simply never see him again. And now—he called her! She was beyond delight. Even if she did harbor that nagging doubt about his remark left in her brain.

In the jail, she asked the clerks, who were always busy with paperwork and questions, "Can I have Clement Johnson's booking records?"

Marie stood waiting, impatient. Medium height, she possessed brown-hair, with huge brown eyes and a slim figure. She had an average look, and people came up to her when she visited other cities and swore they knew her. She would explain that she had never been in Chicago (or wherever) before. Every man who came on to her told her that her eyes were her best feature. She thought so, too. She knew she was no beauty, but she had never had any trouble attracting men.

One of the clerks handed the records over with a shrug. Johnson's records showed that he was arrested immediately after beating his wife severely. The neighbors called the cops, and they arrested him after seeing the condition of his wife's face. Nothing ambiguous about this one.

Marie went back downstairs and consulted with her supervisor.

"Phil, this is a case of deliberate and callous domestic violence. I just don't see any reason for an early out for this guy. Tomorrow is Thanksgiving and I think we should let his family enjoy it without him. We won't help him or them by letting him out early."

"Whatever you think, I agree with you on this one."

Marie then went back to her client. "I'm sorry, but I just can't find a way."

The lady seemed relieved.

"I will tell your husband that you tried your best, but that I was not able to get him out. I spoke to my supervisor about it, and he couldn't see a way, either. I'll explain that to your husband."

At that time, there was no woman's shelter which to refer her. All Marie could do was to give her the phone number for domestic violence help and the woman refused it. Ms. Johnson gathered up her children, thanked her, and left. Marie went back upstairs to tell the wife-beater that unfortunately, he was going to have his Thanksgiving dinner in jail. She told him that his wife had tried her best, but the policies of the court had kept him from being released.

The long day was about to end when Wayne, her favorite cop friend, a sergeant, came in a little after five and said, "It must be five o'clock the day before a holiday."

“Why is that?” Marie asked.

”Because there is a lady lying in the hall calling for a social worker.”

Marie ran to the hall outside their office and found an elderly woman lying on the floor, moaning. Marie bent over her.

“Help me, help me.”

“What’s wrong?”

“I’ve hurt my ankle and I don’t have bus fare.”

Marie said, “If you had bus fare, would your ankle feel better?”

“Oh, yes, ma’am.”

Marie went back inside the office, “Okay, everyone, there’s no emergency,”

She got eighty cents out of her purse and took it to the recumbent woman, who thanked Marie and then got up and toddled off.

Marie sighed and grabbed her purse to get out of there before something else happened. There were few people left in the city jail, most of them had been let out served or through the social workers’ programs or by a judge on time served because they were alcoholics and wanted to go to the Salvation Army’s dinner tomorrow and there wouldn’t be much to worry about. The cops would leave the winos alone this weekend.

Wayne was a cop who tried to live up to the “boy scout” image of a policeman, always trying to help people out. He was dignified, tall, and wore his dark brown hair in a pompadour. Marie had horrified him once when she turned to him in the elevator and blurted, “Is Carla living with you now?”

He turned bright red. Marie had just noticed that he had gained ten pounds and wondered if he was eating better. He answered, “Carla and I plan to be married in a couple of months”. Marie congratulated him and silently berated herself for being so forward. You just couldn't ask Wayne a question like that. He was too private.

He told her the story of his only shooting, when he shot a man who was trying to hold him up while he was in civvies. The victim turned out to be a robber, a rapist, and a murderer. After the shooting Wayne had completely lost it, running up and down the street in the black neighborhood of the City, northeast Oklahoma City, waving his pistol and scaring the residents. Marie laughed and laughed. She knew it wasn't funny, but she couldn't imagine buttoned-down Wayne doing something like that.

When Marie got to the parking lot, she knew where she was going to go. She knew she ought to have more pride, and that hanging with a married man was a loser's game, but the car knew the way to the Bar bar, and she didn't argue with it.

The place was nearly deserted, but Ted was waiting for her. He knew she would show up.

He was rather short, about five feet, eight inches, with curly black hair and dark eyes. He wasn't handsome by any stretch of the imagination, but to her he was the guy she most wanted to see.

"Hi, how ya doing?"

"Oh, I'm fine."

"Well, I'm kinda in a hurry tonight. Will you meet me in twenty minutes?""

"Sure."

He bought her a beer, clasped her hand while no one was looking, and then left the bar. She was to stay in there twenty minutes longer so no one would think they had left together. Then she would go home, and he would be waiting there. Of course, he had his own key so he could let himself in.

In the living room, he didn't even ask about her day. He just said,

"What are we both doing standing around in all our clothes?"

They always yearned for each other, and had extremely satisfying sex, but this night they didn't even have the foreplay of talking about their respective days. They just got out of their clothes and into her bed as fast as they could. The sex was enthusiastic, and they both knew what pleased the other. Sometimes it seemed a little strange that after four years, the sex only got better and better as they tried to please each other more. After the sex, it was a holiday and he needed to get home, so he raced out the door.

Marie went to bed knowing she would have a long weekend ahead of her with her family and no Ted. She wouldn't hear from him until next week, at the earliest. She fell asleep thinking, again, that she was wasting her "best years"—her late twenties, on someone who wouldn't give her anything, but she had no desire to date anyone else. He was all she wanted.

Chapter Two

In the morning Marie awoke, toasted a bagel, and fed Neko. She was sorry to leave her weird Siamese cat, Neko, alone all day even though she wasn't working, but she had to. Neko was her cat for eight years, and the cat loved her even though was extremely unfriendly to everyone else. She bit everyone she came in contact with who tried to touch her, except that she had "gaydar." If a gay guy came into the house, she would leap into his lap and commence to purr. Marie couldn't figure out where she learned that, but she definitely favored gay men. She also believed she owned the neighborhood.

After she had her breakfast, Marie called her mother to see what time they were going to eat and to assure her that she would bring the assigned salad. Her mother, Susie, was a great Southern cook and what she and her sisters contributed meant little toward the preparation of the meal, but her mother appreciated the effort.

Susie was only about four feet, ten inches tall, but she asserted herself and kept her husband and kids in line. She had beautiful, clear blue eyes. Everyone else in the family had brown eyes. When Marie was a child, she thought Susie was the only person in the world with blue eyes, and her mother had the most beautiful eyes in the world.

Both of the grandmothers were Irish, but her father's mother was black Irish. Her mother was the only person Marie knew who had no enemies, and whom everyone liked immediately upon meeting her. She had friends from every walk of life, from the ironing lady she hired years ago, to her friendship with Carol Channing. Marie got impatient with her sometimes over her insistence that her daughters get married and provide grandchildren, but she loved her too much to argue with her. Her mother didn't believe that women should have any interest in a career, because they would just get married and have kids. They should get a degree that would allow them to teach, nurse, or be a secretary, just in case something happened to their husbands.

Marie dreaded the day, for though she loved to be with her mother, her father, Peter, made life difficult. Susie said, "I had problems with my father, too, and I can understand why you all don't get along with him. I know he never seems to approve of anything you do, but he really just wants the best for you."

"Well, mother, why didn't he come to my high school graduation, my college graduation, or when I got my Masters' degree?"

"Education is more important for boys. Girls are just going to get married and have children. He's told you that before. He feels his son is going to carry on his name and he is more important than you girls. He's not right, but you should try to understand how he feels." Somehow, this explanation never satisfied Marie, who believed that her father didn't care about her, but insisted on controlling her.

"Mother, you remember when he wouldn't let me take that scholarship to OU that covered everything, but made me go to that Catholic girl's school that I hated? I had to wait until I was twenty-one to transfer to Oklahoma."

"Your father was afraid you would get pregnant if you went to OU, and nothing anyone could say to him would change his mind. I'm sorry, but that is just the way it was."

Marie sighed as she got into her car. The trip to her parent's house, an old, prairie style home in the Heritage Neighborhood, was short but took her back in time to her childhood. When she went home, Marie always felt inadequate and a little scared, not knowing how things would go. The neighborhood was simply a seedy area of older houses when her father bought this fixer-upper, and he had worked on it for twenty years. Then others got interested in fixing up the classic old houses and suddenly there was a movement to make the area special and thus was born the Heritage Neighborhood.

When she got home, Marie went in the side door. It was always kept unlocked, and every one of the friends and relatives of the family knew it. Her mother hollered, "Who is it?"

"Me."

"You're the first one here. Tim is coming in from San Antonio, Ann's not coming this year because you know how upset Daddy gets with the noise the kids make, and Nancy still is on her way."

She did not mention Shirley, who was in California with her disliked husband, and certainly wouldn't make it home for Thanksgiving.

"Where's Daddy?"

"Oh, he's in the basement working on his model trains. You know him; he won't come up until it is time to eat." Marie frowned.

Daddy had a hobby. He reveled in model railroading, and spent most of his time in the basement workshop, fashioning tiny little buildings for his tiny little town with the tiny little railroad that ran through it. He preferred to stay away from the bustle of food preparation.

Her mother asked, "How's your job going? Are you seeing someone?" Susie wanted to know all about her job and the details of Marie's life.

Marie said, "Well, I had a couple of things happen yesterday," and proceeded to tell her about her domestic violence case and the lady who had no bus fare.

What about a boyfriend?"

"What about it?"

"Are you seeing anyone?"

She didn't mention anything about her reconciliation with Ted; he was a secret from her family since he was married.

"I am not interested in dating right now. That last relationship just did me in for a while," she lied.

Mother said, "We always liked Dex. I don't understand why you didn't marry him."

"It just didn't work out, Mother," she said, lying again.

Marie wasn't about to tell her mother that Dex liked kinky sex and she decided that even though he was intelligent, pleasant, and especially funny, she didn't think she could put up with that for the rest of her life.

"I may not get married at all, Mother."

"But you have to get married and have children."

"No, Mother, I don't."

Just about that time, Tim came in, letting the door slam behind him. "Hi everyone, I'm finally here; boy, what a long drive. How are you all?"

"Fine," answered Mother and Marie.

"Great. I'll just go downstairs and say 'hello' to Daddy."

Tim went downstairs. In the basement, one corner was painted gaily with clouds, mountains, and a pretty waterfall. John, Ann's talented husband, had done the painting. Then a board was added horizontally from the wall, and a town built on it. It was elaborate and had graced the cover of "Model Railroader" magazine.

Their dad jumped up and said, "Shake the hand of an honest man!" How is it going?"

"Pretty good. My classes are going well and I'm all caught up. See, I had time to come up here for the holiday."

Marie went downstairs to speak to Tim. She asked, "Where's Lowell?" Lowell was his roommate of six years.

"He had to go to Minnesota to be with his mother this year, but he will probably come with me for Christmas." Tim was tall, about six feet, and good-looking. He kept himself trim. Of all the members of the family, Marie and Tim looked more like their mother. Everyone else looked like their father.

Marie spoke to her father, briefly, "Hi, how are you," but didn't listen to his answer. He had always been thin, and now had thinning black hair and black eyes, like his mother.

Not only had Tim and Lowell lived together for six years, but also they had moved to two different states together. They were close. Mother called to her, "Hey I need you in the kitchen. I still have a lot of work to do for dinner." As they worked in the old-fashioned kitchen, Nancy came in from El Reno with her new husband, Steve, and joined them in the kitchen while Steve talked with the men in the basement.

Nancy seemed happy and contented in her new marriage, but she, like her mother, was always that way. She was unlike her father and siblings in that nothing seemed to faze her. The three of them quickly prepared the meal and by three o'clock, it was time to eat.

Dinner was always tense. No one knew what kind of mood Daddy would be in. He could be cheerful and talkative, or he might be bitter and angry. If he was the latter, he would pick on one of the kids, usually Marie, who historically, fought back against his barbs more than anyone else, but would be unable to say anything at Thanksgiving Dinner because her mother would be hurt. He would never pick on mother or her brother, and he was generally happy with Nancy.

Marie was happy that dinner went well. Not even their disagreement on politics turned into a fight. Marie asked,

"Who are you voting for this year?" She wasn't surprised when her father said, "Ford."

Marie said, "But why would you vote Republican? Especially after what Nixon pulled and after all those years you voted for Democrats?'

He said, "I just can't trust them anymore. I'm afraid of what they will do to my retirement."

Marie sighed, and didn't say anymore. Her brother immediately changed the subject to his school. "They are starting to make noises about not wanting to employ men who aren't married." Tim taught at a Catholic college, so this could be a real issue for his employment.

Her father noticed that, stating, "That's ridiculous. They'll never do anything like that."

Marie said, holding out her arm to Tim, "Tell them that you married Susan Sullivan while you were in college and you got divorced two years later. Let 'em try to disprove that. Tim looked at her as if she had lost her mind.

Marie used to agree completely with her father about politics—she absorbed her beliefs from him. She was proud of him for being a founding member of one of the largest, most influential unions in the country, but he had recently refused to strike with the other members. He had grown so conservative that he voted for Nixon twice, after she told her mother and him not to do it.

They voted for Kennedy and Johnson; when asked her opinion about Nixon, she told them that it would not be a good idea to vote for him. They did anyway. Marie never said, "I told you so." After her first outburst, Marie was careful to say the right things, though difficult. She had a tendency to just blurt out her opinions and not think of the consequences.

After dinner, she and Nancy helped her mother clear the table and load the dishwasher. They sat around afterwards, catching up with Tim and watching some TV. By six o'clock

Marie was ready to head home. Tim was spending the night, so they wouldn't miss her much. She, Nancy, and Steve said "Goodnight."

Her mother asked if she would be back over tomorrow, and Marie explained, "No, I'm spending the day with Jackie."

"Oh, okay, we'll see you later, then." They were beguiled by Tim's being there and didn't worry too much about her absence.

Chapter Three

Friday Marie slept until 9 a.m., which was late for her. After a quick trip to buy groceries, she called her best friend, Jackie. They were as close as sisters, sometimes sharing the same thought at the same time, and of course, they shared their most secret of secrets.

"Good morning—how's your day?"

"Not ready for prime time," Jackie grumbled. "I'm still un-presentable to the general public."

If I did some housework first would that give you time enough to put on your face and become visible?"

Marie's apartment was messy, as usual, and she hadn't been too concerned about cleaning up. But now she didn't have an excuse. She had lucked into an apartment that was at the end of a row of flats, and consequently was built with an upstairs and downstairs. It had two air conditioners and two heaters and lots of closet space. It was the only apartment like that in the complex.

Marie decorated the downstairs with shiny green wallpaper and put in blinds, and upstairs she hung brown mini-blinds with paper on one wall that had a geometric design of brown, gold and roan. Then she painted the furniture roan. Even Ted was impressed with how good it looked. Marie was proud of it.

An hour later Marie opened the door to Jackie's house without knocking and called, "It's just me."

"Come on in, I'm in the kitchen."

"How's the job going?" Marie asked.

Jackie laughed, "Oh, you know, just one crisis after another. That job will be the death of me"

Years ago, when she was Marie's supervisor at for Child Welfare she always amazed Marie with her confidence and her ability to know what to do in a crisis situation.

Jackie stood six feet tall, was somewhat overweight with dyed black, short haircut and usually wore dangly earrings and way too much makeup. When they first met, Marie thought, Oh, this is never going to work out.

"Marie, I've come up short again this month. Could I borrow $35 from you until I get paid at the end of the month? You know how it is, only getting paid once a month. It's just for food."

"Sure," Marie said. "I'll write you a check. This happens nearly every month, but I know you are good for the loan, and it doesn't bother me to loan you the money."

"Where's Tina?" Marie asked.

"She's with her friends. You know I never know where she is anymore. She's only seventeen but I can't keep up with her. I worry about those friends of hers, and I know she is taking drugs. As you know, twice she has acted so weird I've had to take her to the mental hospital to dry out and it's killing me."

"It must be really been hard on you and on your finances."

"I worry about her all the time. Her father has never been any help."

"Since you are alone, I can tell you all about what happened with Ted this week." Jackie always listened patiently and attentively to stories of her love life. Most people either didn't know, or didn't approve of what Marie was doing, so she didn't have many people to talk with about it.

After they had thoroughly dissected Ted and his problems, Jackie told her about the guy she met who knew his way around the bedroom, but she discovered, "Marie, the man actually voted for George Wallace! Well, I was just horrified.

Can you imagine going to bed with a guy and then discovering that he had those kinds of politics?"

"I guess so. I guess you won't be seeing him again."

"I didn't say that."

They both laughed at that. With their loves lives discussed, Marie decided to go home and get some rest from the weekend before she had to go back to work.

Sunday afternoon she finished a book in the afternoon, and decided to see if there was anything on TV. It startled her when she turned on the set and saw downtown Oklahoma City, with a newsman exclaiming, "The riot is almost under control now, with the crowd dispersed and several people arrested." Marie gasped and covered her mouth in horror. "However, the police did not come out in force during the entire incident."

Marie ran to the phone and called her office. Wayne answered the phone,

"Oklahoma City Police Department, Officer Wayne Brixton, Community Division, how can I help you?"

"Wayne, what in the world is going on? Do you need me to come down and help with the phones?"

"No, you would just get in the way. It has been a horrible afternoon and we are still not sure what happened. You stay home now and I'll see you tomorrow."

Marie continued to watch as the newsmen showed the scenes of chaos over and over, with young men throwing garbage cans and rocks through the windows of John A. Brown's and Rothchild's and the other stores up and down Main Street, looting and destroying what they could not carry away.

The rioters were Hispanics. Marie saw few policemen and wondered why. She could only watch in horror with the rest of the people in the City, and wait to find out what happened the next day.

Monday morning when she went to work, many patrolmen were holding shotguns, one in front of the door to her section's office. She touched his shoulder and asked, "Is it safe to go in?"

The policeman answered laconically, "I'll make sure it is."

She went in and immediately starting asking questions, but couldn't get any clear answers.

"What happened yesterday?" She asked Wayne.

"It was Saturday night. I don't know any details, but a cop killed a kid, a Hispanic one. So the Hispanics held a rally yesterday, and it got out of hand. The Chief thought, given the circumstances, the police ought to keep a low profile, so quite a bit of damage was done. I don't know any more."

"You don't know how the kid got killed?'

"I've heard some rumors, but nothing definite. We'll just have to wait."

She worked all day in the tension-filled department. When she asked questions, the answer was always the same, "I can't speculate, and what I know I can't talk about. Besides, you aren't sworn. I can't tell you anything."

One of her friends, Gary, said, "I picked up a kid who flagged me down. He was badly cut and needed stitches. I took him to the emergency room, and while I was waiting for the young man to be treated, I watched TV. I was not too surprised to see that kid, on tape, throwing a garbage can through the window of the John A. Brown Department Store. So we came straight back here and he wound up in City Jail."

Nothing happened all day. It was quiet at the police department and on the streets. It seemed that the rioting was all over with, but its cause was still a mystery to Marie.

Finally, around four p.m., the boss called a meeting. When Marie took the job with the Police Department, she was dubious about working with cops. However, the Community Group, the section she worked in, had surprisingly caring employees. The best part was the boss, Harry, who had movie-star good looks, with dimples, blue eyes, and lots of brown hair, was one of the most intelligent men she'd ever met, and really knew how to handle employees well. She loved working for him and considered him the best boss she had ever had.

One morning Harry, who was always the first in the office and the last to leave, met her at the coffee pot and said, "You know, I really appreciate the way you come in early and stay until the job is done."

Another time Marie made a bad miscalculation and managed to run out of gas on her way to work at eight a.m. on the access road to the freeway. Harry sent a patrolman with gas to rescue. When she got into the office, he said sternly, "We are not here to fuck it up. Don't do that again." It was never mentioned again.

The worst mistake she made with Harry was the time a patrolman asked for help and she told him she couldn't help because of a doctor's appointment. Marie actually hoped to run into Ted at the Bar bar before the appointment and was reluctant to spend the time to help the cop. The patrolman complained to Harry and he had a talk with Marie, saying, "We can't leave the patrolman in the lurch when he needs us."

"I agree. Harry and I made a thoughtless mistake. It won't happen again."

Again, Harry dropped the subject.

Today, Harry started off the meeting by saying, "I don't want you to be in the dark about what happened, or to have to speculate. Let me be clear, you can tell anyone what I am going to tell you. Saturday night, a burglary took place in a service station, in which a vending machine was broken into and some change stolen.

One of the patrolmen, Officer Brown, along with his partner, Officer Wokin, picked up a couple of Hispanic kids, twelve and thirteen, who were known troublemakers. They took them out of their beds in the middle of the night, and questioned them in the patrol car. When they denied any knowledge of the burglary, Office Brown decided to play Russian roulette with the thirteen-year-old kid to try to scare him into a confession. The officer thought he took out all his bullets, but he missed one. When he spun the barrel and pulled the trigger, he shot the boy in the head with a .357 Magnum." There was a gasp from the listeners, and comments like,"How could he be so stupid?" and "Why would he do such a thing?"

Marie was suddenly nauseous and the implications of such a terrible action started to hit her.

Harry responded, "I think he was inspired by a movie, and got carried away. Of course, he killed the boy, and he immediately jumped out the car and tried to shoot himself, but he was out of bullets. As he was fumbling in his pocket to find bullets to reload with, his partner was able to overcome him. Then he cuffed Brown and called for an ambulance and his supervisor. The chief ultimately gave the news to the children's mother, but you can't make that right. On top of that, they took fingerprints from the vending machines, and they did not match the kids, so they had nothing to do with it.

Don't be reluctant to tell people the truth, because as bad as it is, it is better than lying or just telling them part of the facts. This is terrible, but the truth needs to be out there."

Harry dismissed them, and all of them expressed their shock to each other, but wanted to get away. Marie headed for the Bar, excited, but horrified to have news to pass on to Ted and her friends.

Chapter Four

It took a minute for her eyes to adjust to the darkness of the bar, but then she saw the biggest table surrounded by the newsmen who frequented the place. Ted, even though he wasn't a newsman anymore, was there too.

When she asked him, "Why did you give up your job on the radio?"

He said, "Well, I won best radio newsman in the country last year and best radio news story. I thought I couldn't top that, so I decided to go into public relations for a while."

The newsmen greeted her noisily and pulled up a chair for her.

"Marie, tell us, what happened?"

Marie told them what Harry just told their work group.

Glenn said, "I had heard some of it, but not all the details. Wow, what a story."

Tony exclaimed, "I'm glad you came in. We needed to hear that."

Marie replied, "I knew you would be here waiting to hear what I knew."

Buddy asked, "Where were the cops during the riot?"

"The chief thought it best that the cops stay out of the way and just let the riot wind down; He thought that their presence would just add fuel to the fire."

"Can we report that?"

"Sure, you can report anything I've said."

The conversation continued, pretty much in the same vein. Ted was too much into it to go home with her. Marie had to come back to work the next morning and, since it had been such a slow day, thought it might be busy tomorrow.

"Goodnight, guys," Marie said. They absentmindedly chorused a faint "Bye," and she left to go home.

In the next two weeks, things slowly got back to normal at work. A couple of days later, Wayne came in after lunch and remarked to everyone in the room, "I just went to the bank to deposit my check. People looked at me like I was a baby-killer. I'm not wearing this uniform again until Brown is in the pen."

And he didn't.

Public opinion surprised Marie. Radio talk shows and letters to the editor were completely against the way the Chief had handled the riot. Marie thought it was the prudent thing to do, but the public seemed to think that the police should have been out in force, shooting and arresting the looters.

"Wayne, what do you think about the way the Chief handled the riot?"

"I agree with the Chief and the way he handled it, but I think most cops believe he handled it wrong. We may see some fallout from this."

Marie was upset, because she liked this Chief. Whenever he saw her, he'd say, "What are you doing?" He listened to her answer and either tell her "Good job," or make a suggestion. He was interested in all his troops.

A few days later, she was surprised to get a call from Ted at work. This time, he greeted her and then asked, "Have you heard anything about the P.R. campaign the Community Office is gearing up to put on?"

"No, just that they have been working on it. I'm not involved with it."

"Well, can you find anything out? My agency put in a bid and we are worried about it. Marie said, "Okay, I'll see what I can find out."

Marie didn't have a clue how to find out what he needed to know. If Harry were asked, he would tell her she didn't have a need to know, as would anyone else she tried to get the information from. "You know, we don't want the information to leak before it is released."

Marie worked until after quitting time. Sure enough, Harry went off to a meeting after five. She didn't know where he had gone or how long he would be, but took the chance to slip into his office. The report on the project and how the different agencies ranked lay on his desk. She grabbed it and ran to a copy machine; slipped the copy into an envelope and addressed it to Ted at his job. She managed to get the original back on Harry's desk before he returned.

Two mornings later, Marie was surprised to see Ted in Harry's office. She said, "Hi, do you two want coffee?"

They both said, "No," and went back to their discussion. It wasn't until Ted came over to her apartment that night that he said, "That report you sent me showed our agency in last place. I went in this morning to try to undo the damage, but I'm afraid it didn't work."

"Ted, I guess that was the worst thing I have ever done. I can't believe I took that report from Harry's desk. He always tells me what a good employee I am and how much he trusts me; and look what I did."

"Well, you did it for me so it doesn't matter. Besides, you didn't get caught, so it's okay."

They ate the barbeque Ted had brought; a little remained for Neko. They took the time to have some special and tender sex, which always pleasured both of them. Then stoned, they watched "Monty Python's Flying Circus" on PBS. Marie didn't have her contacts in, so Ted tried to describe the action on TV to her. It made them both laugh so hard they were weak. Ted left around two a.m., so it would be a late morning tomorrow, but at least it was Friday. Marie still felt bad about swiping the report.

Saturday was routine, with chores and shopping, until she got a frantic phone call from Jackie in the evening. "Marie, Marie, the cops were here!"

"What happened, Jackie?"

"You know that guy I didn't like who was hanging around with Tina?"

"Yeah, I remember."

"The son of a bitch was an undercover cop and he has been giving her drugs. You know she has flipped out twice and I've had to send her to the mental hospital to straighten up—well he is the one who supplied her. He gave her drugs for free and she couldn't handle them."

"Oh no! What happened tonight?"

"He came over with a bunch of other cops with a search warrant and an arrest warrant. They tore my house up but didn't find anything."

"Oh my God! What are you going to do?"

"Well, the first thing I did was call Larry. I am so glad you referred me to him. He's a smart lawyer. He said that if I can get her back to the Vespers, the mental hospital, before the cops get to her, he can keep her out of jail."

"How can you going to do that?"

"I've talked to her on the phone and told her not to come home. She is hanging out with the street kids on Tenth. She needs a ride to the hospital and I can't do it. I may be watched by the cops."

"What are you going to do?"

"I am counting on you."

"Jackie, you know what will happen to me if I am stopped with a kid who has a warrant on her in my car."

"I know, Marie, but I really need you to do this. You are the only person I have to help me."

Marie reluctantly agreed to the plan. Jackie said she would get word to Tina to call her at home and tell her where to pick her up. Marie hoped that it would work out without her intervention. However, a few nights later, she picked up her phone to hear Tina telling her she was ready to go to Vespers.

"Can you pick me up?" Tina asked

"Where are you? Marie got directions and headed over to the "hippie" part of town.

When she got to the designated location, Tina paced on the corner. She got into the car and to Marie's surprise, seemed subdued and respectful.

"Tina, do you know you have nearly worried your mother to death? Do you know how close you came to going to jail?"

"Yes, I know, and I'm really sorry."

"Tina, this is really important. If the cops, or anyone, ask you how you got to the hospital, tell them you hitched. Do not, whatever happens, tell them that I picked you up and took you there. It would mean my job if it got out. And do you know how lucky you are they agreed to allow you to come back after that scene you created last time?"

"Yeah, my mom told me that. Don't worry, I won't tell anyone you picked me up."

"I could get in trouble for it."

"Okay, okay."

Marie dropped her at the hospital and hurried home, grateful that she hadn't been stopped for anything. She didn't know how she could explain that to Harry.

Chapter Five

Marie stopped hearing from Ted. She waited for a call every weekend, but it never came. She spent a time with Jackie trying to make her feel better about Tina's situation, and with her family, but always home at night, waiting for the phone to ring. On the third Saturday night she didn't hear from him, she went to the Bar bar. He was there, but he was with a woman she didn't know. He ignored her completely, and she pretended to ignore him.

Marie sat at the bar, chain-smoking cigarettes, adding to the smokiness of the bar. He was in a booth with the woman, who was not particularly attractive with short blond hair and was about ten years older than Marie. Marie indicated by her closed-in body language that she didn't want to be bothered in the mostly-male bar so no one spoke to her. She couldn't hear what Ted and the woman were saying, but could tell by his animated countenance that he was charming her.

She left after a half hour, but parked her car in the parking lot next door, and sat for two hours just to watch them leave together. She wanted to be sure that they did leave together, and that it wasn't just paranoia. While wrapped in her car blanket in the cold, she was hurt and dismayed that he would make moves on a woman while she was in the room and that it didn't even bother him to hurt her like that. She thought about their relationship and knew that she yearned for him. Her father had not loved her and she would naturally try to win the love of a man who wasn't capable of loving her. Still she sat there, in the dark and the cold, until he came out of the bar, after two hours, holding hands with the blonde. They both got into his car and drove away.

Tearfully Marie returned home and paced the floor in her cowboy boots all night. She didn't sleep or eat at all until Sunday night. She always knew that he cheated, but now she had seen it and that reality made it twice as hard to take. She was frantic that she would lose him now.

After several weeks, she became more receptive to Nick, the city planner who had been coming on to her for a while. They had met at work, though they didn't work in the same department. She had fallen into conversation with him because she had once had a notion to study city planning.

Nick commented, "This snow is just right. It didn't mess up the streets too bad and it looks pretty. I'd love to have someone to cuddle up to tonight."

Marie was lonely and looking for someone, so she said, "I'd like for you to come over tonight. It's Friday evening, so we don't have to worry about time. I think there is a good movie on TV. I'm in the apartments on twenty-second and Douglas that are kind of old-looking, Apartment 623."

When Nick arrived he was dressed in a reindeer sweater, wearing glasses, and with short, curly hair.

"So, Nick, how is the job going?

"Pretty well, how about you."

"I like working for the City and I enjoy the variety of the job, however, it is a dead end for me. I once started a graduate program for city planning but didn't follow through."

"That's a shame," Nick replied. "I'm sure you would have been good at it.'

After a decent amount of small talk, he made a move and they decided to go to bed. However, it only took a few minutes for Marie to realize that this wasn't going to work out for her. He made love to what was rather, to her, a violent fashion and she couldn't seem to calm him down. He was hurting her.

After she had decided to just get through it, the phone by the bed rang. Marie knew only one person who would be calling at eight on a Friday evening. She grabbed the phone, and said warily, "Hello."

Ted answered, "Hey, what's going on over there?"

"Nothing much, it's pretty quiet." Nothing was going to keep her from seeing Ted.

"How about if I come over?"

"No problem."

Marie hung up the phone and turned to Nick, "You have to get dressed and get out of her now! That was my boyfriend and he said he was coming right over—and he has his own key. He'll be here in five minutes." She started to push him out of bed.

She made it sound as though it were a dangerous situation rather than an embarrassing one. Nick flung on his clothes except for his shoes and socks, while Marie jumped in the shower and then found a robe. She said a hasty "Good night" to him as he dashed out the door, then emptied ashtrays and tried to straighten the place up. It was looking pretty normal when Ted arrived.

She was suspicious from the way Ted asked what was happening and the way he checked out her apartment when he got there that her neighbor, who was eighteen and had been flirting with him, had tipped him off.

Nick later told her he was sitting in the snow in the parking lot putting on his socks and shoes in the snow when Ted drove up, but Ted didn't see him. That was the extent of her relationship with Nick. It embarrassed her, but she and Ted went ahead to have sex with their usual enthusiasm. Nothing, it seemed, could keep her from enjoying herself with Ted.

The next morning her neighbor passed her on the way to the parking lot and said, "You're running them in and out pretty fast now, aren't you?"

Marie was too embarrassed to answer as he walked off, chuckling. Her face blushed red.

Chapter Six

Marie noticed new tension among the cops at work but no one was talking, not even Wayne. There was a story in the newspaper about a man who showed a police ID to a woman, gained entry to her apartment by asking "I need to watch the apartment across the way. Can I use your apartment to do it?"

The woman agreed and he asked to use her bathroom, then emerged naked and raped her. The police department put out a warning for women to watch out for this man who was impersonating a police officer, but still it happened twice more.

The Daily Oklahoman kept printing the warnings, "If you are confronted by a man with a police ID, call the police department and ask if the policeman has such an assignment."

Marie didn't realize it, but the reason for the tension within the department was the fear it was a rogue cop who was doing the crimes. It came to a head. The man confronted a woman, who happened to be one of his fiancé's friends. After he raped her, she said, "I know who you are. I helped Felicia order that custom shirt you're wearing."

The policeman who had used his real ID to get in, and his service revolver to threaten her, then shot her through the eye. Assuming he had killed her, he left. However, she later regained consciousness and called for help. She identified the rapist. It was none other than Oliver, a policeman in Marie's division. She knew him well, and knew that he was a lady's man, but he had never turned his charm on her. Wayne told her, "I sort of expected it, but it is still hard to believe. I knew he was strange."

This situation didn't endear the citizens of Oklahoma City to the police chief. The chief had become more unpopular with some of the cops and certainly with the citizens as the latest embarrassment rolled out, but mostly they were still unhappy about the lack of police response at the riot.

The City Council, after much discussion and input from the citizens, fired the chief and the whole police department underwent a shake-up. Harry was promoted to Assistant Chief in the Traffic Division, and Ed, a Captain in patrol, would become their new Director in Harry's place. It upset everyone, but Marie went to Wayne almost in tears "What am I going to do? I don't know if I can work for anyone but Harry."

"He's been promoted to Assistant Chief, and we'll get a new Director. I don't know much about Ed, but we'll just have to get along with him."

"You know, Wayne," Marie said, "Everyone has been pushing me to join the force. I have a good excuse not to, because my vision is so poor and I have to wear contacts. However, the truth of the matter is that I'm not sure of my judgment when called on to make a split-second decision. I won't ever feel like one of the troops if I don't get sworn."

"Judgment is the hardest part of being a cop, and if you can't be sure of yourself, you shouldn't try," Wayne said.

A few days later, Ed, introduced himself to them. Harry had given them a nice "goodbye" speech, in which he said, "I'll be taking over the Traffic Division, which is a big job." He added, jokingly, "And I'll finally be able to get those jaywalkers, who are my pet peeve."

Afterward, he took Marie aside and said," I couldn't say this before, because it would have been sexual harassment, but

I'm not your boss anymore. If you ever get lonely, just call me."

Marie was taken aback, but didn't reject the idea. She hugged him good-bye. She had always been impressed by Harry, almost to the point of idol-worship while he thought her attractive.

Ed didn't seem to be enthusiastic about their mission of community service. He just seemed to be happy to have been promoted. The first time he said something to Marie; he dragged her over the window and pointed down to the sidewalk.

"Look at that!" Have you ever seen anything that bad before?"

The only thing Marie saw was a mixed-race couple walking down the street, so she answered, "What? I don't see anything."

He pointed again. "There, by the alley."

Marie said, "No, I can't see anything" and turned away.

Wayne walked from the water cooler, took her aside and told her she should have gone along with the Director's prejudices, because now he would be unhappy with her.

Marie sighed. "Wayne, I am in a dead-end job with a boss who already doesn't like me and I don't like him. I can't transfer under Harry because there aren't any civilians in Traffic. I just can't take this. I can't work in a place where I'll never be promoted and the boss is a racist."

Marie immediately sat down and wrote out her resignation letter, giving two weeks' notice. She had no idea where she would find a job, but Marie didn't like the direction this workplace was going in.

She had her exit review with Harry in his new office, which was much bigger and busier than the last one. He commanded hundreds of employees now and would not be the first person to work and the last to leave at night anymore.

"I gave you a good review with a recommendation for rehires should you ever want to return to the City. I hope you find something you like soon. I enjoyed working with you."

With that, her police department career was over, and Marie was unemployed. She took her retirement, because it would give her a few thousand to live on while she looked for work.

Marie started job-hunting immediately, but came up empty. She had a Master's Degree and a teaching certificate and ever since she graduated she tried to get a teaching job at the high school level, but with no success.

Finally, someone told her, "We don't hire people with MAs because we have to pay them a thousand extra."

It made her both depressed and angry, because it was difficult for a woman to get into graduate school and to obtain a graduate degree at the time she did it. Now it counted against her.

Marie picked up some part-time work in the local junior college, but it was little money. Certainly not enough to live on. They paid her a thousand a semester per course taught. Most of the teachers were part-timers, so there was little chance to get on full-time.

She worked part-time and tried to get a job as a teacher or social worker. Marie really wanted to be a writer, and had wanted to be one since she learned to read, but didn't know how to break into the field. With no experience, when tried to write her mind went all over the place. That was frustrating, wanting to write but not being able to organize herself.

After several interviews, she talked with Jackie. "Jackie, I am really getting scared. I've interviewed five times but no jobs and I'm about to run out of money. My teaching stipend won't even pay the rent, and I'll soon move in with you."

"We can't have that. I'll tell you what--Food Stamps is hiring right now and I'll bet I can get you a job right away there."

"What?" After what happened with Child Welfare?" Why, they wouldn't even look at me."

"No, it's a different group of people and if I gave you a good recommendation you could get in."

"Oh, please, Jackie, if you are able to get me a job you can forget all about that $125 you borrowed from me to help pay Tina's bills. Marie threw her arms around Jackie and hugged her.

The next day, Jackie called and told her where to go for her appointment with a Food Stamp Supervisor. Marie eagerly put on her best clothes, made herself up, and reported at the time specified. She wasn't excited about the idea of giving out food stamps, but it was better to be on the giving end rather than the receiving one.

The office was in an abandoned shopping mall, drab and dreary; painted olive and light green. Marie wondered if the government was still using paint it bought during WWII.

When it came time for the interview, it was another "this is never going to work out" moment. The boss was obese, at least 400 pounds, and wore his hair in a pageboy. While he was neat and clean, that cute little haircut made him look like Tweedledee.

"This job is really pretty basic," Don said, "you just interview people and determine from their answers and paperwork if they are eligible to receive food stamps." He assured her that she would receive more than adequate training, and then said, "I don't know if you know this, but the state pays only once a month."

"Oh, yes, I know that, but it won't be a problem." Marie knew that from her year at Child Welfare, and she knew it was going to be tight.

"Well, I think you'll do well in the job. Just report here next Monday at nine."

"Thank you. I appreciate it. I'll do a good job for you."

Marie drove home, not excited about the job, but glad to have one. She called Jackie immediately, and told her. "Jackie, guess what! We did it. I'm employed again. I start next Monday."

"I just didn't want you to move in here. I've got enough on my plate with Tina," Jackie said, laughing.

Chapter Seven

Marie trained for her new job. At first, it seemed complicated, but soon it started to make sense and she realized the rules were so rigid and demanding that each interview with every separate client would be essentially the same. That made her feel more secure in starting a new job. The biggest problem was that the feds set the standards and the state funded the program. She could see a clash coming between those two mandates.

When her training was done, she was assigned to an office that served a predominately black neighborhood. About half of the workers were black, a few were Hispanic, and the rest were white. Everyone seemed to work together well. Her first interviews were as she thought they would be, with most of the clients eager to please so they could get their benefits. However, the workload was heavy, nine interviews a day and nine cases to work up and fill out forms to be entered into the computers. The forms had to be filled out perfectly or they were returned; then the stamps had to be issued by hand, which was a long, drawn-out process. One day a week was "duty day" when a worker was assigned desk duty, catching all the walk-ins and emergencies. It was hard at first, but Marie learned to work fast, and Don was a helpful supervisor.

One of her first interviews was with a Hispanic family with a man, a woman, and three small children. She asked for identification, and the woman gave her a driver's license and birth certificates for the children. The man offered nothing. Marie asked, "Don't you have any ID?

"No," he said, "I am from Mexico."

"How about a green card?" Marie asked.

"No, I don't have a green card, "he said.

"So you are not here legally."

"No."

"Well, you are not eligible for food stamps, but I will look at your income to see if your family is. Your income counts even if you aren't eligible. Is there any income in the house except yours?"

"No."

"Do you have check stubs?"

"Here."

Marie calculated his monthly income and found that he made too much for the family to be eligible for benefits. She explained the problem to them and denied their application. The next time Marie saw Don, she asked if there was anything special to be done with this case. He said, "I need a carbon copy of a form 9907 showing that you have reported the man to the INS."

"But Don, that makes no sense; this guy is supporting a woman and three kids. It would be crazy to deport him."

"I said I needed a carbon copy of form 9907 in the file. That's all," Don repeated,

"Oh." Marie was learning the ways of bureaucracy.

Meanwhile, Ted had been coming over more often, about twice a week. Every time he came he brought marijuana. Marie always had a hard time sleeping. After discovering how well she slept after smoking marijuana, she found a small-time dealer in her apartment complex and starting smoking every night.

One night he arrived early and they immediately lit a joint. After half an hour, they were as stoned as people can get on marijuana. They ate the dinner Ted brought, and he stripped down to his jockeys to lie in bed and watch television.

Suddenly, "Your antenna is not aligned right," he said.

"The antenna is fine. Don't worry about it."

"No, it's not right. I've got to fix it."

"Ted, it's on the roof. You can't fix it. Just relax."

"No, I'm going to fix it. Where is your screwdriver?"

"I can't remember. I know I have one somewhere. Let me think."

"No, I'll just use a knife."

Ted got up and went to the kitchen and found a good-sized knife. He then went to the sliding glass door that led to the balcony and opened it.

"Ted, you can't climb up on the roof! You'll fall. And you're in your jockey shorts. Please don't do it."

"I can hold the knife in my teeth and everything will be fine as long as nobody calls the police."

"And what if someone does? They'll report a man in his underwear on the roof, with a knife between his teeth. That won't be good."

"You'll back me up that I was just adjusting the antenna."

With that, Ted climbed up on the balcony rail and pulled himself up on the roof. Every few minutes he would holler, "is it better this way?"

All Marie could do was giggle uncontrollably and yell back the status of the TV until the adjustment was better. He was happy with what he did, but the next time it rained, Marie had a leak right over her bed. She feigned ignorance when the maintenance man asked her about the antenna.

"It's not mine; it was here when I moved in. I just hooked up my TV to it." He looked dubious, but seemed to take her word for it.

Monday night Ted called her early in the evening. "Guess what? Sheila left me this weekend."

Marie suddenly felt light-headed and had to grab the wall for support. It had never occurred to her that something could happen to Ted's marriage. He had never discussed it with her, and she never asked any questions. Now, she thought optimistically, Ted will spend his time with me and won't feel the need to run around.

He invited himself over, and this time brought a change of clothes. "You know, I don't have to pay tuition for my wife any more, and I just have myself to support. I want to get back into the news business and move back into the area near downtown, but I need a little help to make the transition. Can I stay with you for a few weeks until I can make this happen?"

"Oh, that's a great idea. I know you love news casting and this will be a real opportunity for you. I'd be happy for you to stay here." Of course, Marie was thrilled that he would be around her place.

After he spent the night, she noticed that he swung his feet out of bed and immediately smoked a joint. Marie needed her morning cigarette, but didn't want to smoke marijuana in the morning. She thought it was a little odd, but of course didn't want to irritate him, so she didn't remark on it.

When he left for work, he said, "I'll give my notice and will probably be fired immediately. So it may be only a few days until I am back with my stuff."

"Okay."

Marie went to work on a cloud, and told her new friend, Bobbie, all about the good news. Barbara was a slender redhead who had been in the same training class with her and was now working in her unit. She had told Marie all about leaving her husband for her current husband, whom she met on a vacation. Bobbie and Marie were becoming close friends.

All that week Marie was excited and walking on air. On Friday night, she decided to visit Shirley, who had recently moved from San Jose to Bethany, a suburb of Oklahoma City. Shirley had recently gotten a divorce. She never voiced any of the details of her marriage to anyone, but everyone in the family suspected the marriage to Brent was not good.

Marie was planning to spend the weekend with Shirley and the kids. As she was heading to her apartment, she saw two young men hitchhiking on the street. She stopped and picked them up. "We are from Oklahoma University and we want to spend the weekend in the City, but we don't have any place to stay."

Marie was so pleased with the way her life was going that she decided to help the guys out. "I am going to be out of town this weekend, so you can use my apartment. I went to OU and know how you can need money. I'll drop you off there and when you leave, you can just push in the lock in the door handle. Oh, and don't try to play with the cat. She'll bite you."

After she dropped them off, she drove to Shirley's house and spent the weekend with her, helping her to decorate her new house and getting re-acquainted with her nephews Brent, Jr., and Sandy. Shirley took after Daddy's side of the family, so she was five ten, with dark hair and an olive cast to her skin. Sandy and Ben, Jr., were also tall for their ages, but that wasn't surprising since Brent was six-six. They also had lighter hair and skin.

She was happy to be with her sister and what was happening at her apartment never crossed her mind.

Marie and Shirley talked about marriage. After hearing Shirley's stories, Marie said, "I was pretty sure I never wanted to give up my independence to get married, and now I know it. It just isn't worth it."

She was happy to be with her sister and what was happening at her apartment never crossed her mind.

Chapter Eight

Marie returned home late on Sunday afternoon. At first, she was puzzled by the dirty dishes in the kitchen and the note on the table by the door. Then she remembered the hitchhikers and felt a sudden stab of fear. She checked the house and found everything intact. The guys had only eaten some food and slept in the beds. Both exhaling with relief and realizing how lucky she was, she read the hand-scrawled note thanked her for her hospitality and telling her they had a good time clubbing in the City at Fuzzy's and two other clubs, and then left Sunday morning.

Oh well, she told herself, it would turn out all right. They said they were from OU. Besides, I'm a great judge of character. She knew what it was like to be broke in college and was glad to help them out.

Monday she went back to work, still waiting to hear from Ted. He didn't call until the weekend and he showed up with a suitcase.

"I had to get the lease settled, and the furniture split up, and all that good stuff. However, the divorce has been filed and we have taken care of the worst part. I'm just going to miss the cat. If Neko weren't such a fighter I would have tried to keep her, but I know your cat wouldn't tolerate her."

Within the first week, they fell into a routine. Marie went to work about seven-thirty, while Ted networked on the phone with his old friends from news stations. She noted when he got up in the morning he either took a hit of speed or smoked a joint, and she wondered how he chose what to take. She thought it odd, but didn't say anything. Ted took drugs, but he was not strung out on them. He also drank an amount that Marie thought was excessive. However, he was never arrested for driving under the influence. He just seemed to need the drugs and alcohol to function.

At night, he stayed out late drinking beer and playing pool. Between midnight and two a.m., when the bars closed, he'd call and wake her up and ask her what she wanted to eat. She'd answer, "A chocolate shake," because that was all she could handle at that time of night, and he would get himself some fast food. When he came home, they would eat, smoke, watch some late-night TV, make love, and go to sleep.

She finally figured out he must be napping in the afternoon; otherwise she didn't see how he could keep up such a schedule. During the second week, he came home early one night, and started pacing the floor. He wasn't communicative, and it took her a while to divine what was wrong. Then, she pulled a twenty out of her purse and said, "Do you want to go play?"

"Yes, I do. I hate to take your money but I feel all cooped up. I'll pay you back when I start working."

At some point, she told him about the hitchhikers. "Oh, for god's sake, don't be doing that. I don't care how innocent they look, I don't even care if they are women, many of them are ex-cons or criminals or rapists and you are risking your life."

"But I like meeting new people and helping them out."

"Listen to me. Don't ever do that again. Period."

"Okay, "she agreed, reluctantly.

~*~

One evening he came home early. "Looks like a big storm coming our way."

"Yes, I was glad to get home before it rained."

In a few moments, they heard the first thunder crack. They grabbed bowls of ice cream, ran upstairs and got into bed, after raising the blinds over the big window by the bed. Marie turned on the TV and muted it. They watched the lightning and listened to the thunder, awed by the majesty of it all. After a quarter of an hour, the rain came bucketing down: it simply poured. Both of them were used to this kind of weather and considered it a form of entertainment.

After the first hour, though, things got ominous. The sky took on a greenish cast, the rain let up, and the clouds above them started to rotate. By this time, Ted was listening intently to the television and told Marie, "I've got to call in."

Marie wasn't surprised. She also wasn't surprised when he said, "I have to go now. I don't know when I'll be back. Don't wait up."

He had been interviewing with a station and volunteered to go in and help. They were used to violent storms in the City. The only time Marie actually saw a twister, she was coming home from work and was on an elevated highway when she saw a perfectly white and beautiful-looking twister in the sky. It had not touched down yet so it was still clean.

She couldn't do anything, so she just stared at it. She took the first exit and headed for shelter, but she never forgot the strange beauty of it. After all the storms, she went through in the City, that was the closest a tornado ever came to her.

At the end of the second week, Ted landed this newscaster job at one of the largest radio stations in town. It would be a couple of weeks before he got paid, but he was working again, and in a job he really liked. His spirits improved, but his hours didn't. He seemed happy to work drive time, but he still stayed out until the bars closed.

When he staggered home, Marie asked him, "Are you drunk?"

"If I'm not, I just wasted thirteen beers."

He borrowed his spending money from Marie, asking her to keep track of it until he was able to accumulate some cash. Still, he didn't spend a lot.

After another three weeks, he found a nice apartment pretty close to Marie's and moved in. After being with her for so long, he stopped calling and coming around. She had been so happy while he was staying with her it was a shock when he dropped her.

While riding the bus back from a trip downtown one Saturday, a big, good-looking guy sat next to her. Marie often took the bus when she went downtown because she didn't have to deal with parking. This guy was about six feet, six inches tall, blond, and had blue eyes. His name was Charley.

He started joking with Marie and soon had her in stitches. He was so funny that the people around her were laughing with them. At the end of the line, Charley asked for her phone number and she gave it to him. The next day, he called, "Hey, can I come over and see you?"

"Sure," Marie said. He lived close so it didn't take him long. They were in bed in no time, and afterwards he said, "You know, I am married. My wife and I are real happy right now because she just had a baby."

"Well, what are you doing here? Seems like you ought to be at home."

"It's kind of nerve-wracking at home at times. Sometimes I just like to get out and forget my problems and laugh."

"I thought you said you were happy with the new baby and all."

"I am, but something happened five years ago and it is scary."

"What happened?"

"I came home from work one day and my wife had killed our four kids. Strangled them with my neckties. They were all lined up on the bed."

Marie sat up in bed, surprised and flummoxed. “Oh my God, Charley. That is terrible. What happened?”

“They sent her to a mental hospital and she was let out a couple of years ago. It’s only been now that we have had the nerve to have another child,” Charley said.

“I think you better leave now and go home and be with your wife and child. And I don’t think you should come back here. I don’t want to be involved with you—you need to spend all your energy and time with your wife,” Marie said. “If anything happened, I would think it was partly my fault and I don’t want to go there.

Charley left then, but not too happily. Marie was upset; even her stomach was feeling bad. The first thing she did after he left was to call Jackie.

“Jackie, you aren’t going to believe what just happened to me. Let me tell you.”

Jackie was horrified when she heard the story but found it as hard to believe as Marie had. Marie wasn’t sure she believed it entirely, but she didn’t want to be around anyone who told a story like that anyway.

The next evening, after work, Marie got a phone call from Jackie. She said, “Marie, you aren’t going to believe the referral I got today.”

“What was it?”

“It was to open a case on a guy whose wife had killed his kids five years ago and they have just had another child. So your guy wasn’t lying yesterday. It is hard to believe.”

“Oh, Jackie, I am so sorry I ever met the guy.”

Marie felt bad for a long time over that one-night stand. She swore she would be more careful in the future and stop letting guys just pick her up.

At work, her supervisor, Don, was promoted and Marie got a new boss. The new supervisor was a black woman who changed Marie’s job from an in-house interviewer to a new-applicant interviewer. A new applicant got a home visit, which required that Marie make seven home visits in a day. These were scheduled by clerks, who did not take into account where the applicants lived, so the routes made no sense.

Marie couldn't work up the cases in the field, so she had to take them home and fill out all the paperwork at the house. Marie had to do it daily or get way behind. She was never good at finding places, so looking for addresses was hard for her. However, after a few months, she knew the neighborhood well.

At home, she got the feeling that the neighbors were avoiding her. She didn't think much of it, being busy with the job. She barely noticed that a new bar, the Turquoise Lounge, opened at the end of her block. She had stopped going to the Bar bar since she didn't have to meet Ted anymore; he was free to see her any time he wanted. Marie really wasn't much of a bar person, anyway. Finally, her next-door neighbor let her know that Ted was hanging out in the evenings at the Turquoise, and he was spending his nights with Janice, an eighteen year-old girl who lived in Marie's complex.

Marie had only talked to Janice a couple of times and had found that they had nothing in common. She read only romance novels, left her curtains open at all times, even when she was in her pajamas, and talked constantly about her "daddy," who, from what Marie gathered, she adored. The thought of 40 year-old Ted sleeping with Janice made a shiver run down her back.

She was hurt and upset. My god, the girl only lived three doors from her. This time, she called Ted,

"Ted, as long as you find it necessary to date Janice don't come back around me."

"You can't tell me who to see."

"All right, then."

This time it really was over. She couldn't believe he would dump her, after seven years, over a child. An uneducated one, at that.

Marie cried all night but dragged herself to work the next morning. She didn't call in sick because she only did that when actually sick, and she wanted to talk this over with Bobbie. She hadn't called Jackie because her friend had so much trouble right now, but she was bursting to talk about this development with a woman friend and to gain some sympathy. Marie was desolate.

Chapter Nine

Bobbie listened to Marie, agreed with her that Ted had acted badly, and then tried to convince her that she would be better off without him.

"After all, Marie, he never took you out, never introduced you to his friends, and ran around on you. And with your neighbor, no less."

"But I love him and I didn't want to give him up. I will miss him terribly. It's just that I couldn't ignore his running around with Janice."

"Of course you couldn't. You'll get over him in time. Now let's get to work."

Marie felt awful, but she got through it. She thought Ted would come back.

But he didn't. Marie sat by the phone every night. She wished she could afford an answering machine so she could go out and leave her phone alone. Marie went out on the weekends, to see her family and Jackie because she knew if he called it would be late. But he didn't.

She hadn't seen Ted and Janice together at all for about two months. One nice afternoon she was sitting in her living room doing her paperwork with the door open, hoping that a neighbor would come by and chat. To her surprise, Janice wandered into her apartment.

"Hey, how are you?" she asked.

"I'm fine."

"What are you doing?"

"Just doing some paperwork for the job."

"Would you believe that Ted two-timed me?"

"Really, sorry, but I have to get this work done. Can't talk now." Marie waved her arms vaguely.

She was astonished that Janice would come to her for sympathy, but she sure wasn't going to give her any. Marie didn't say more because she simply didn't want to talk to her at all.

Another neighbor, Lynda, who was recently separated from her husband, decided that both she and Marie needed a night out and talked Marie into going to a club with her. She wasn't too enthusiastic but was bored sitting at home so much of the time. They went to this raucous rock club with a live band. It was an open-air club with people sitting in the bleachers in the hot summer air. The people were young and jeans-clad.

As they were sitting watching, others come in, Marie saw a guy come in the door and said, "Oh, Lynda, look at him. The one with the blond hair. I hope he comes this way!" She lost him in the crowd, but started a few minutes later when he sat down next to her.

"Hi, I'm Marie," she yelled.

"My name's Wilson," he hollered back.

"What do you do, Wilson?"

"What did you say? I can't hear you."

"I said, what do you do?"

"I work for the electric company. I check meters when people have a complaint about them. And what do you do?" He responded. Marie barely heard him. She answered, yelling,

"I give out Food Stamps."

"Let's get out of here. It's too loud." She excused herself to Lynda and Marie and Wilson walked to her apartment down a deserted street, which was mixed business and residential. It was only a few blocks to her apartment. As she opened the door, she gave her usual warning to new people, "Hey, don't pet the cat, she bites." Neko, after all these years, barely tolerated Ted except when he brought her food.

To Marie's great surprise, Neko jumped in Wilson's lap and demanded petting as soon as he sat down. Now, Marie knew what that meant generally, but she just couldn't be right about Wilson. Why would he bother with her if he were gay? So she pushed the information out of her head.

They spent that evening just talking and Marie liked him a lot. Maybe, she thought, she really had found someone who could take Ted's place. They stayed up most of the night before he left, and when he did leave, he took her phone number. Marie's depression lifted quite a bit, and she felt much better at work the next week. Thursday night Wilson called.

"Hey, you want to come over Saturday and have dinner?"

"Sure. Where do you live?"

"I live out by Lake Hefner," he said and gave her the address and directions.

"I know where that is. See you Saturday night."

After they hung up, she made a run for the drawer where she kept her map and figured out the route. It was a long way, but it was worth it.

Saturday night she put on a new pants outfit and her makeup and headed out about six. She wanted him to think that she dressed up for him—she didn't just slap on some jeans and a t-shirt, but she really wasn't completely sure of her motivation to seduce him.

It took her over half an hour to find his address, but she did find it, with a little trouble. Marie was directionally challenged. When she finally pulled into the driveway and got out of the car, a little black and white dog ran up to her. She started petting it and it jumped up in delight.

Just about then Wilson came out of the front door. "That's Zig-zag. I want to show you what he likes to do."

"Okay."

With that, Wilson pulled a branch from a large tree down to the ground. Zigzag grabbed the branch in his mouth and Wilson let go. Zigzag was pulled up in the air about six feet. He then began to gyrate, and soon was swinging in circles. Marie couldn't help it, she laughed uncontrollably at the little dog whirling in the tree. After a few minutes, Wilson lowered him to the ground and he barked and jumped around.

"I've never seen anything so cute in my life. Why does he do that?"

"He loves the attention. He'll do it until you stop laughing at him. I don't want to wear him out though; it's hot out here. Let's go inside."

The house was a little brick one, but as she stepped inside but it was surprising to see he had not picked up before she got there. The house was clean, but there were several items scattered about, and when she excused herself to go to the restroom his work clothes were laying on the floor. The kitchen was all-white, devoid of any decorations.

Oh well, she thought, he's just a man, he's doing pretty well.

Wilson called out for pizza and while they ate, they talked about work. He explained to her what checking on meters that people complained about entailed and told her about the time he smoked marijuana before he went to work. "I left all my keys hanging in the door of a meter box at a children's playground and didn't realize it for fifteen minutes. I decided not to smoke on the job again."

Marie gave him the basics about food stamps, then told him, "I was at the home of this really dignified black minister when the elastic on my slip decided to let go. Right in the middle of my interview, my slip fell down around my ankles. Unfortunately, he didn't think it was funny so it was hard to pull it off."

Wilson laughed at that with her. About this time, they mutually decided to go to bed. At first, it seemed all right, but then it became clear that he only wanted only anal sex and she wasn't willing to do that. He kept pushing her to do it, and she kept saying, "No."

"If you won't do what I want then you might as well leave." Marie found her clothes and slipped into them, then, as politely as she could, said goodnight. Her heart was pounding and she was a little afraid of him. By the time, she got outside to the car she was seething, remembering now that Neko had told her that he was gay and she had ignored what the cat was communicating to her. Marie didn't know if he were gay or just kinky, but she didn't want to go back there in any case.

Now she had to drive home in an unfamiliar neighborhood in the dark. She was shaky about the route and kept guessing at the turns. She was scared and upset. Finally, she got to a main road and knew her way from there. She had planned on spending the night there. Dammit, this was a ruined night and a wasted date, and she was for sure going to miss Zigzag.

Chapter Ten

Marie's date with Wilson made her gun-shy about going out with anyone new. She missed Ted even more. Coming home from running errands the next Saturday, she drove to Ted's apartment without planning it. She wasn't dressed up or even made up. She just wanted to see him so badly that it was sort of on automatic. As she pulled around the corner of the complex, she saw him looking at her from his open front door. By the time she got parked, he disappeared.

Marie knocked on his door, not knowing if he would answer it or what she would say if he did. He opened the door, "What are you doing here?"

Marie had to say something, so she asked, "Where is the money you owe me? It's been three months and I haven't seen a penny of it."

"Dammit, I haven't paid you because I haven't got it. I'll pay you the money as soon as I get it."

"Wow," Marie said as a distraction, "What a nice apartment."

"I know. It has taken all my money to pay the deposit and rent and to get it furnished."

The apartment looked out on a little lily pond through huge windows. It was at the end of a quiet cul-de-sac. Inside, it was modern with stainless steel accessories and Ted had furnished it accordingly with a stainless steel and glass coffee and end tables. He had neutral couch with nubby fabric and had hung interesting pictures around the room.

Ted and Marie stood and looked at each other awkwardly for a few minutes, neither one knowing what to say after three months apart and the way they broke up. Finally, Ted said, "Say, what are we doing standing around with all our clothes on?"

"Gee, I don't know," Marie answered.

They went to bed and found that they hadn't lost a step in three months. The sex was just as good as it had ever been, tender and yet exciting. They both put all their effort into it to make it good.

Afterwards, Ted said, "I'm sorry, but I can't let you stay. You know tomorrow is Mother's Day, and my mom is in town and I promised her I would take her out to eat tonight. I'll have to ask you to go pretty soon so I can get ready."

Somehow, it didn't sound completely right to Marie, but why should he lie to her? They had just made up in a big way and everything was fine. Marie chose to believe that his mother really was in town, though she had never known her to visit the City from Kansas before.

"Okay. Listen, just out of curiosity, how did you get Janice to go out with you after she knew you were staying with me?"

"Oh, I told her that you and I were just friends and that you let me stay with you because I was broke and needed a favor."

"And she believed that?"

He laughed. "She was lousy in bed, not bright, and talked constantly about her father. I wouldn't have been interested in her except that she is eighteen and I am forty-two."

"Well, I could do the same, but oddly enough, I wouldn't be interested because, guess what? Young guys are lousy in bed."

Ted laughed at her and told her it was time to go. "I'll call you."

She left, walking on air. When she got home, feeling better than she had in months, she decided to go over to Jackie's house since she had the evening free and hadn't seen her in a while. She bathed and put on clean clothes and stepped out her door into the courtyard.

However, she couldn't have been more surprised. There was Ted, walking toward her. She thought he was coming to see her and, with a big smile on her face, she took a step to meet him.

He grimaced and motioned her away. Then she saw him knock on Janice's door. She quickly dove back inside so she wouldn't have to see any more. She went upstairs, flung herself on her bed and cried. He was planning to see Janice the whole afternoon he was with her. And that story about his mother! Okay, this time she was finished.

Instead of going to Jackie's she decided to stay home and feel sorry for herself. She sat in the living room in the dark and cried. Ted and Janice went past her window toward her apartment about eleven. She got up and closed the curtains, mad at herself that they had even possibly seen her. Right after that, though, she heard Ted walk by her apartment to the parking lot. Well, he hadn't spent a lot of time with her.

Marie was sure she wanted nothing more to do with Ted when he called her next day. A phone call from him was the last thing she expected. She experienced real surprise and joy when he apologized, said, "I already had a date set up with Janice, but that was the last time I'll go out with her, please don't stop seeing me."

Marie said she would continue dating him, "If he never got his apartment doors mixed up again."

"Okay, I promise."

For a while, he saw her regularly and seemed to ignore Janice. Then as was his habit, he disappeared. Marie started keeping track of when he was calling her and when he wasn't, and, after a time, discovered a pattern. Generally speaking, he was seeing her for about three weeks and then made himself scarce for six weeks. She had no idea what it meant.

In the next few weeks, Marie saw Ted in a green car with a woman whose main physical features were that she looked almost identical to Marie. It was funny, because two of Ted's friends told her she was a dead ringer for Sheila, his ex-wife. Even Marie could see the resemblance between her and the new girl. She never learned her name and though she could have followed him and learned where the girl lived, Marie decided that Ted wasn't going to leave her anyway, no matter how many girlfriends he had. It was eight years since they had started their affair, and he was still coming around. She decided to stop worrying about it.

One morning that fall, she woke up and turned on the radio to hear Ted give the news and weather. That was, of course, the first thing she always did while she had her first cigarette of the day. He reported the news and then promised a beautiful day with a high of 65, so Marie went off to work without even taking her coat. It was sunny in the morning, but got cloudy later and went she went outside at five o'clock to go home from work Marie was surprised by cold temperatures and snow flurries.

She headed home, glad that her car heater worked. Just when she got downtown, well into a construction zone, one of her tires blew on the interstate. Marie pulled to the shoulder and sat in the car, not knowing what to do next. Not close to a phone, the only thing to do was to wait for a patrol car. After an eternity, a man stopped his pickup and offered help. Marie opened the window only a few inches and handed him her mechanic's card. "Please call this gas station and ask them to send out the service truck to change my tire. I don't think I even have a jack." "Sure," he said cheerfully, and drove off.

About a quarter of an hour later, the man returned. “I called your service station and they said their service truck is broken down. I’ll take you to the station to borrow their jack.”

Marie sighed. It was snowing and dark-thirty. The choice was to freeze to death or take a chance on getting raped. She got out of the car, said “Thanks” to the man and they checked her trunk. She couldn’t remember who had changed her tire last, but, as she suspected, she didn’t have a jack.

So then, she made an even greater leap of faith and got into the man’s truck. Marie had always had good luck in letting me help her with broken-down cars, and it seemed like it was going to work out this time, too. But it was so scary, depending on a stranger and getting into his car, knowing you were taking your life into your hands.

He said, “I’m Bobby.” He was a pleasant-looking cowboy who was balding. He drove her to the station, borrowed their jack, and took her back to her car. He changed the tire, but had to do it in ankle-deep mud. After all this, he said, “Will you go out to dinner with me?” Marie didn’t particularly want to; she just wanted to go home and get warm but thought it would be churlish to refuse, so she said, “sure, I’d love to.”

At dinner, Marie warmed up and began to feel better. Bobby said, “I’m from Weatherford. I’m in the oil business. I’m in the City for business and I come back here every so often. Can I call you when I am here?”

Marie, warily, “Are you married?”

“Yes, I am, he replied, “but my wife and I are separated and are getting a divorce.”

“Sure, then, you can call me.”

They parted, with Marie saying, “Thank you, thank you for stopping and helping me, again; I want to thank you for stopping. Not everyone would have done that. I really appreciate that. I don’t know how long I would have been out there in the cold and the snow. I just can't tell you how much I appreciate it."

The phone rang when she stepped inside the door. Marie said to Ted, "Boy, that was a lousy weather report you gave this morning," she said.

"I don't make them, the Weather Bureau does that; I just read them," he replied.

"Today I went to work without a coat because you said it would be warm. I nearly froze when I blew a tire on 35. Some nice man stopped and helped me out, or I would still be there."

"Well, you should listen to me for updates during the day," he answered.

"Sorry, I can't do that. Can't do interviews and listen to the radio."

The next morning at work she spoke to her friend, Doyle, who was in the office adjacent to hers. Doyle was tall and thin, like Bobby he was balding, and he was younger than Marie. She knew he was from Weatherford, in fact, he had just moved to the City before he took this job. She told him about her adventure, and asked if he knew Bobby.

"Sure I know him. I've known him for years."

"Is he really separated from his wife?"

"I don't think so. He and his wife have seven children and as far as I know they are getting along fine." Doyle answered.

"Just my luck again."

Chapter Eleven

That winter, Ted lost his job. He had to give up his apartment and move in with Marie again. That was fine with Marie; she loved having him around. This time it was a little harder for him to find a job. He finally had to take one as a news director for a radio station. He didn't mind the extra money, but he didn't want to deal with a budget or with hiring and firing. Ted said, "Anyone who gives me a hundred thousand dollar budget to fool around with is an idiot." Ted just liked to get out there in the field and report the news.

One night while they were in bed talking, Ted said, "You know, I'd have to be a slow learner to get married more than once. But I can see you married with a whole passel of kids."

"Ted, what a horrible thought. No, I don't ever want to get married. I value my independence and my freedom to spend my money and my time the way I want to. You'll never catch me getting married."

"We'll see."

It was a colder than usual winter and it snowed a lot. Marie was scared of driving in the snow and ice, and Doyle picked up her up in his four-wheel drive vehicle whenever it was slippery. Of course, Ted always went to work, no matter what, because if he didn't, there'd be three hours of "dead air" on the radio and he needed to tell people about road conditions. A couple of times that winter he came in from de-icing his car to say, "You aren't going to work today."

Sure enough, Doyle called in a few minutes to tell her that driving wasn't safe that day. She hated missing appointments, because it threw her schedule off. However, everyone in the City had their schedules thrown off because of the weather, and the clients missed appointments, too, unless they were in walking distance of the office.

Marie never spent a holiday with Ted. Since he was staying with her, she thought they might actually enjoy the holidays together this year, but Ted went home to Kansas to spend Christmas with his family. Marie spent it with her family. She was disappointed, but there was still New Year's.

But when New Year's Eve came around, Ted asked,"What are you going to do on New Year's?"

"I've been invited to a party by someone I work with," answered Marie, hoping that he would want to come along. She didn't want to tell him that she was not planning on going without him, because that would sound somewhat pitiful.

"Good, because I plan to get together with some guys and play poker."

Marie was disappointed that he didn't want to come to the party with her or that he didn't make another suggestion, but pretended to be cool with her plans. It meant that Marie had to go to the party, but she did like the woman who was giving it, Lois, who was a worker in her unit.

It was cold the night of the party, so Marie put on tights, a long blue flowered skirt, and a blue silk turtleneck. She had a good time. Lois invited people from her church, her Peace Corps group, her husband's work, and her job, so there were a lot of people to meet and talk with.

Marie was a little down because Ted hadn't wanted to do something with her, and she drank a too much. Marie did not drink much generally, because she and alcohol did not have a good relationship. When she drank even a small amount, she had a tendency to fall asleep. This time she lay down on the Lois' white couch right after midnight and passed out. About four-thirty, Lois shook her and said,

"Marie, it's time for you to get up and go home." Marie, embarrassed, found her coat and took her leave of the few people who were still there. She was happy about one thing, though. She had been determined to stay out longer than Ted, and she was sure she had succeeded.

When she got home, Ted wasn't there. Marie was chagrined that she had beaten him home. He didn't roll in until about six o'clock. He said, "I had a great time playing poker. Lost everything I had."

"I just got home. The party was great. Too bad you couldn't make it."

It was so late they just went to bed and slept late. When she did wake up on New Year's Day, Marie felt funny. It was hard for her to breathe and her face felt weird. She got up to look in the mirror and was shocked to see what she looked like. Her face was swollen; he eyes were nearly shut and her cheeks were even with her nose. She looked strange. Her stomach was upset, too.

Marie knew what it was. She picked up the phone and called Lois, who thankfully was already up. "Lois, that was a great party last night. I really enjoyed it, thanks for inviting me. Listen, this is kind of awkward to ask, but did you clean your couch before the party?"

Lois gasped, "Oh my God, I totally forgot you're allergic to cleaning fluid. How is it?"

"Pretty bad. I'm all swollen with hives. I'll have to get to doctor before I can come to work."

"Oh, Marie, I am so sorry I should have known better."

"Lois, you can't be expected to remember everybody's allergies. Don't worry about it."

Since it was a holiday, Marie couldn't do much except lie there and feel bad. Ted got more and more uncomfortable, and finally made a decision.

"I can tell you don't feel well, and I am just in the way, so I'll go to Anthony's house for a couple of days until you feel better.'

Not up to argument, Marie said "good-by" weakly and watched him pack and go. She felt abandoned just when she needed help. She didn't feel like she could ever count on Ted for anything.

She didn't call her family for help because they did not approve of her relationship with Ted. They thought she gave in too much and he got away with too much. Therefore, they didn't know the details of what went on or even when he was staying with her.

After three days in bed, Marie felt better and decided not to take time for the doctor, she just went back to work. She was still embarrassingly swollen, but she felt well enough to work. That night Ted called, and asked, "How are you doing?"

"Well, I'm back at work so I'm feeling better."

"Okay, I'll come home tonight."

He did come back, and everything went on as usual.

Ironically, two weeks later, Marie was surprised to hear his key in the door just after she got home from work. She went to the top of the staircase, and asked, "What are you doing home so early?"

"Oh, I've caught the most awful cold or the flu. I'll have to go straight to bed."

He crawled under the covers with a box of tissues and started watching television. Marie said, "What do you want to eat?"

"I don't think I want anything. I feel terrible."

"You have to have something. You'll never get well if you don't eat. Try to think of something you could eat."

"I don't know," he answered. He thought for a while. "How about some cream of mushroom soup with oyster crackers?"

"I'll have to go to the store, but I'll get them for you. Just try to rest."

Marie went out in the cold, irked because he certainly hadn't tried to feed her or make her feel better when she was ill. She got even more upset when she had to go to three stores to find oyster crackers. She wondered why there was an oyster cracker shortage all of a sudden. Marie finally got it together and returned home.

"Okay, Ted, I got your dinner."

"Hey, I thought of what I really want while you were out."

"What do you mean, what you really want?"

"Well, I decided I didn't want soup and crackers, what I really want is frozen Sara Lee cheesecake."

"Okay," she said, and she didn't think she sounded patient at all when she said it.

She knew better than to pitch a fit—that would only upset him and he would leave. She didn't want that to happen. So she gritted her teeth, put her coat back on, and went outside, slamming her car door as she got back in.

There was a grocery store right across the street and luckily, they had the cheesecake. Marie bought two just to be safe. When she got home, his craving hadn't changed again, so he happily sat in bed and ate.

He stayed home from work for three days until his voice sounded better. Marie had already bought him enough food for him to get by, but she had to get cold medicine for him, too. She didn't allow herself to show any anger, and he was happy to let her care for him while he convalesced.

Chapter Twelve

Ted moved out of Marie's apartment when he was able to get another apartment. He also made a new friend, Charles, who was the disk jockey during drive time when it was Ted's shift to deliver the news.

One night in February, Marie became upset with Ted over something (she couldn't remember what later) and went to his apartment and pounded on his door. Charles was there.

Ted said, "Whatever problem you have, we'll have to talk about it later, I'm busy right now."

Thus dismissed, Marie went home pissed off. She stopped at her neighbor Eric's house to tell him her troubles. He was a medical student who had only lived in the complex for about a year. They had started a close friendship.

"Did you know that "Easy Rider" is going to be on TV tonight? I want to watch it because I've never seen it."

"I've never seen it either," Eric said. "Why don't I come over after I finish my studying?

"Okay, it comes on at ten."

Marie went home, but she was still too upset with Ted to work up her cases for the day. She decided to set her alarm for four a.m. and get up early to do them. She smoked some marijuana to calm herself, remembered that she hadn't locked the front door, and then thought it was all right because Eric was coming over soon. She dozed off.

Marie was confused when she was startled awake by the alarm. She realized she had to work on her cases, but still she hit the snooze button. As she was rolling over to snatch a few more z's, she thought she saw Ted in her apartment, and that puzzled her. Then she realized it was not Ted.

A man dressed in black, looking sinister, was bent over doing something on the floor. Marie had a loaded gun, but it was in the drawer of her bedside table—no time to get it. The man walked toward her, and she finally made out what he was holding in his hand. A knife. Marie imagined herself being raped and killed. She thought, *I don't want to die like that.* She sat up and screamed.

He walked passed her and toward the stairs. Marie grabbed the phone and dialed the operator and said,

"Give me the police," just like in the movies.

While she told the police operator there was a man in her house, she grabbed her gun out of the drawer. She put down the phone (not going to put down the pistol) to slip on a nightgown, prompting the operator to shout, "Hello, Hello? What are you doing? Are you okay?"

Marie shouted back, "I'm fine, I'm getting dressed."

But the operator couldn't hear her and she had to juggle the phone and the pistol to reassure her.

Two cops, guns drawn, kicked open her front door and came in. Marie went to the top of the stairs, her .22 in hand, and told them she thought the man was gone. They told her to put her gun down. When she didn't respond, one of them came up the stairs and pried the pistol out of her shaking hand. He said, "Let's go into the bedroom so you can get more clothes on and show us what he took."

Marie went over to the spot where she first saw the man, and said, "Oh, that's why he had a knife." The antenna cord to her TV had been cut. The policeman looked where she pointed, while the other one looked into her open bedside drawer, still hanging open where she kept her pistol and a lid of marijuana.

Marie's heart dropped and she held her breath. Oh, no. I had to go through all that and now I'll have to go to jail!

The cop did not do a double take or indicate in any way that he saw the marijuana. Neko was under the bed, crying, and the patrolman crawled under the bed and grabbed her to make certain that she was all right. Marie didn't have time to warn him, but luckily, Neko was so scared she didn't bite him, either.

About that time, the snooze alarm on the clock went off, startling everybody. Marie got her robe on and went downstairs to check on the rest of the house. The cops had decided not to call out forensics when she told them the burglar had on gloves.

She told them, "He was black, dressed all in black, and he looked really scary. I can't say any more because I didn't have my contacts in."

She checked the kitchen and the living room and discovered that her cash was missing, all twelve dollars of it. She was still shaken, and the policemen were nice, but they couldn't stay with her until it got light and she calmed down. They asked her if there was a neighbor they could get for her.

"Please," she said, "ask Eric, next door, to come and talk with me until dawn."

So they went next door and knocked on Erik's door. Marie had forgotten something, though. Eric had a closet full of gro-lights and marijuana plants. When he saw two policemen at his front door at five a.m., he nearly went into a panic himself. He was polite while the policemen were there, but after they left, "Marie," he said angrily, "How could you frighten me like that? You knew I would be really scared to see policemen at my door in the middle of the night."

Marie answered, "I know, and I am sorry. I wasn't thinking about your plants, just about how shaken I am. Please stay here until it gets light. Oh, and why didn't you come over last night?"

"I studied late and forgot all about the movie."

"That's the last time I'll leave the door unlocked for you."

"That's probably a good idea," Eric said.

After about half an hour, when the sun came up and Marie had calmed down, she worked up her cases and got ready for work. Then she remembered she had no money for lunch or cigarettes. She took a detour on her way to work and dropped by Jackie's office.

When Marie saw her, she exclaimed, "Jackie, I had a burglar last night and he stole all my money. Can I borrow ten dollars?

"That's terrible. Of course, you can. Call me and tell me all about it tonight." Jackie was busy and Marie needed to get to work, so it was a fast transaction. When she got to work, Marie told everyone about it and they sympathized with her. She felt fine but tired all day, and wasn't shaky until she got home. When she did, she checked all the closets and the space between the wall and the refrigerator and under the bed and thought about calling Ted to come over and spend the night. She told herself to get over it and she might as well start now.

Late that night, after she had told Jackie the whole story, the phone rang and it was Ted. "Hey, Charles and I are over here, and I want you to come over and watch TV with us."

"No, Ted, I had a burglar last night and he scared me so much I don't want to come out in the dark. You two come over here."

"No, we're too drunk to drive over there. Just jump in your car and drive over to my apartment. It's not that far."

"No, Ted, "said Marie, "I don't want to. I'll see you some other time.'

Marie had already smoked marijuana, so she was in no shape to drive and really was afraid of the dark so soon after her scare. She fell asleep, but soon woke up gasping and sweating. Marie had dreamed the man was back and leaned over her bed. She came awake with a jolt. She finally realized why the man looked so scary. Besides his all-black attire, he also had on a black ski mask, with white rings around his eyes and mouth.

The next day Marie called one of the policemen who responded to her call and told him about her dream. "Now I can't even be certain of the race of the guy, since he was wearing a mask."

The policeman said, "The chances are slim to none that we will ever catch him, you know that."

"Yes, I do." Marie said, "But thanks for being so understanding with me that night."

Over the next few days, Marie got over her fright, but her gun was not kept in the drawer any more. She swore that no one would ever make her feel so helpless again, and she moved the gun to side of her bed, between the mattress and the side of the bed, so she just had to let her hand drop to grasp it. It was kept there from then on. She also wore a nightgown every night after that one, kept a robe on the foot of the bed, and bought a pair of glasses so she could see the next burglar. She also figured that things would go much better in the future if she kept the door locked.

Chapter Thirteen

Marie started feeling better about her life. She liked working for Bobbie, who had been promoted to supervisor, and she came back into the office to work instead of doing home visits. She decided not to worry about Ted anymore, and did quite well with that. One night as lying in bed, almost asleep, she thought she heard him walk by her apartment, but didn't even rise up from bed to look out her window to see if it truly was Ted.

The next morning, when she opened the blinds to let the sunshine in, she couldn't miss his car parked on the street right under her balcony. Marie shrugged her shoulders and got ready for work. It was never mentioned to him. She didn't worry about where he was when he wasn't around; she just thought it was nice when he was. She wondered, though, and not for the first time, if good sex was enough to keep a man around for ten years. Would he have stayed so long if he didn't care for her a little? Maybe she was too available and made it too easy for him. But Marie couldn't bring herself to ever say "no" to him, she didn't want to upset him, and didn't want to miss an opportunity to see him.

Just when it seemed things were going well, to Marie's great surprise and distress, Charles found both himself and Ted an out-of-town job and they both quit their jobs and went for it. Both of them put their belongings in storage.

Marie didn't know until she heard him talking to Charles on the phone about plane tickets. Infuriated, she did something she had never done before. When he hung up the telephone, she confronted him angrily. "You were talking to him about plane tickets for the day after tomorrow. You were just going to leave town and not tell me. I can't believe you were going to do that to me!"

Ted said, "No, I wasn't, but I'm not going to sit here and listen to this."

With that, he got up and left.

Marie was hysterical. She had never talked to him like that before, and he had never walked out on her before. She grabbed up all his belongings and threw them in a pile on the bedroom floor cursing and crying. Just about the time she was calming down, he came back into the apartment. "Hey, I just wanted to…"

Then he saw his stuff. He silently gathered it all up and left. Marie just stood there and cried.

For the next three weeks, she didn't hear from him, then, to her surprise, he called and said that he was coming home. He was caught in the middle of a strike at a radio station, with each side expecting him to take their side.

He did come home in about a week, and nothing was said about their fight.

In a few weeks, Ted and Charles got another job. Hired as a team, they were to set up radio stations in different towns using preprogrammed tape and didn't need personnel, just engineers. This time, Ted said, "goodbye," and "I don't know exactly where I am going, so you can't contact me, and I don't know how long I'll be gone."

Marie was devastated, but she kept a stiff upper lip and hugged him goodbye. She didn't cry or show her feelings of dismay to him. They made love as if they never would again, and then he left. He was so looking forward to his new job and life that it didn't seem to occur to him that Marie was bereft, and she went along with the idea.

And with that, he was gone. Marie fell into a depression, not knowing if he would ever come back. For the first few weeks, she only went to visit her family when her mother called and asked her to, and seldom visited Jackie, since she was still monopolized by her problems with Tina. It seemed easier to just stay home.

After a while, she returned to the Bar bar, to meet men. One of them would ask, "how are you doing?'

And she would answer, "Fine." She had no problem picking him up for the evening. This happened two or three times, but didn't make her happy. Then she started calling Harry, "How are you doing, big Assistant Police Chief?" she'd ask.

He'd say, "I'm really busy now, but I can come over and see you Wednesday after work."

Marie still missed Ted and wondered constantly where he was and what he was doing.

She would wake up in the morning and make a couple of pieces of toast with her coffee, but she could never get down more than half a piece. She never felt hungry. She didn't have a scale but could see she was steadily losing weight. When she got dressed for work she'd look in the mirror and she'd note that it looked like she was wearing her older sister's clothes, but she didn't care.

One day when she got into work, Bobbie was talking to her over coffee and said, "You need to go for some counseling. You are losing weight and obviously unhappy; you are letting Ted dominate your life even when he is gone."

Marie knew that something wasn't quite right, so she agreed to go to the Mental Health Clinic.

She set up an appointment. The Clinic was a small, squat brick building close to downtown where several bus lines converged. Inside, it was dingy. They set her up for weekly counseling sessions, with the fee based on her income. The psychologist assigned to Marie had tried to brighten up his office with an Oriental rug.

The counselor listened to her story. "I am in love with a man who does not return my feelings and who has left town with evidently no problem in leaving me."

"How does that make you feel?" asked the counselor."

"It makes me feel bad, it make me wonder why I wasn't good enough for him."

"What do you do with your time?'

"I work at Food Stamps. It keeps me busy during the day, but at night I mostly sit at home and don't do anything."

"You should try to get out more," said the counselor.

"Yes, I know I should, but I am depressed; I've lost about twenty pounds and I don't feel like being around people."

"You know, you are young, attractive, and intelligent. There is no reason for you to be depressed. You just need to stop it. Don't be depressed anymore."

Marie asked him, "How do I stop being depressed?"

"Just don't do it. Get over it. Just stop."

Marie went back for three weeks, only to get the same advice each time. Then she just stopped going to counseling. She couldn't see that she was getting any help. Marie was quite capable of telling herself to not to be depressed, but it didn't work. There was logic in what he said, but just telling herself not to be depressed did not elevate her mood.

Thanksgiving she went to San Antonio, to her brother Tim's home to celebrate with her parents, her brother, his friend, and Paul, her mother's brother. Their family had never really had good Thanksgiving memories.

One of her father's sisters, Aunt Chloe, had traditionally hosted a huge feast for her friends and family every year and they were expected to attend. Her father especially disliked going there and his unhappiness rubbed off on the rest of the family. Everyone dreaded Thanksgiving. The food was served buffet-style and you ate where you could perch. However, as Aunt Chloe got older, she was unable to throw a big bash each year and the family tentatively started making new traditions.

As soon Marie she arrived in her brother's and his partner's stucco, Mexican-style home, and said her "Hellos," her mother immediately drew her aside to one of the bedrooms. Her mother was upset and Marie had seldom seen that. Her mother was always an island of calm in their household and their world. She was so upset she was shaking. Marie asked her what was wrong, and she answered, "Daddy wants me to get plastic surgery, and I don't want to."

"What! Why would you get plastic surgery?"

"Well, he says I have gotten so old and wrinkled he can't stand to look at me anymore and I need to have plastic surgery to look better. He says I am not pretty anymore like I was when he married me."

Marie scoffed, "You don't need plastic surgery. You look fine."

"I went to a doctor and he said that my skin was too thin for a facelift, so I went to Merle Norman and had a makeover. He still isn't happy with me."

"Mother, you tell him to go straight to hell. He has no business telling you to get plastic surgery. He hasn't gotten any younger and he's not so great to look at. He's losing his hair, and even though he's always been thin, he's getting a paunch now, and he has plenty of wrinkles himself. Don't let him bother you."

Marie helped her brother with dinner, fixing the salad and helping with the vegetables, but the big turkey was Tim's job. He did a great job with it even though he was nervous about it. Marie stayed in the kitchen with her mother and brother to avoid her father as much as possible. It was all she could do to be icily polite to him.

Tim's hobby was collecting fine china and crystal and the table was beautiful. He had obtained a lace tablecloth like her mother always liked to use and ordered some fresh fall flowers. He really tried to make it a memorable occasion.

They ate dinner and, since no one else knew how her mother felt, it went off fairly well. Mother was not going to ruin the occasion for Tim and Lowell, the hosts, and wouldn't argue with Daddy in public. She was also conscious of Paul, her mother's brother, being there and she always put on a good face for him. Marie was simmering. This treatment of her mother was ridiculous and she was angry at the thought of it. It was obvious it had hurt her mother.

Sitting in the living room after dinner, her father was upset that only Marie and Tim had shown up, even though Tim had knocked himself out putting on the dinner. He whined to his brother-in-law, "You know, my children never loved me."

Marie spoke up immediately, saying, "You had to love us first."

Then, angry and fearing she had started a scene; she got her things and stormed out. Paul was visibly horrified at the way she was talking to her father. Because her uncle was there, she didn't say more, but when she got home, she called Tim to apologize for leaving abruptly and leaving him with a situation.

Tim was confused, "I never noticed that anything was wrong; nobody said a word about it."

Marie told him what mother told her; Susie hadn't told him about it.

When mother got home, Marie called her and talked to her again about Daddy wanting her to have surgery. "Mother, this is all in daddy's head and there is nothing wrong with you. Don't let him intimidate you. I am going to lay low for a few weeks, but call me whenever you want to. I feel really bad that he has tried to make you feel bad about the way you look. Please don't worry about it."

"Okay," she said, I'll call you when I get upset about it. You're the only one I have told and I am embarrassed to tell anyone else. Let's just keep it between us..."

"He'll get off on some other tangent after a while. Just ignore it."

"Okay," she said.

Marie was still furious, but knew there was nothing she could do to change her father's attitude. She couldn't believe he did that to a woman he was married to for forty-six years, but she knew her mother wouldn't leave him, either. Her kids had wished for years that she would leave him, but she had signed on for life.

Chapter Fourteen

Marie soldiered on, going to work every day and trying, but not succeeding at, keeping her spirits up. Just when she thought it couldn't get any worse, Jackie called.

"Marie, I know we haven't talked much lately, but I have something to tell you. You know how I told you my periods were all messed up and I thought it was stress. Well, I finally went to the doctor, and she says it is cancer."

"Oh, Jackie, no. How bad is it?"

"Inoperable and terminal. I have only a few months."

"Jackie, that can't be right. You are so young. You've never seemed sick to me. I can't believe it."

Jackie said, "It is not easy for me to believe, either, but I have had to accept it. I haven't told many people yet but I thought you should know. I feel pretty good right now but I have to start chemo next week.

"I hope it isn't too bad."

"I'm afraid I will lose my hair that really scares me. I don't want that to happen."

"I promise I'll help you any way I can, but I really don't know what to do." Marie didn't know how to convey her feelings.

"Call me and let me know."

When she called Jackie back to see how she was doing a few days later, Jackie said, "I had my first chemo treatment this week and it made me so sick! I threw up for three days.

Wanda suggested I try smoking or eating marijuana next time before the treatment, but I don't want to model that for Tina."

"Well, maybe you should, Jackie."

"No, I am just going to stop. I was just buying time with it and I don't want that kind of time. I just want to make it until Tina graduates from high school. I hope I can hang on that long."

Ted was gone, and now she was losing the person she could always count on, the one who had been there for her for the last decade through everything. It never occurred to her that she would lose Jackie. Jackie was young, only thirty-nine years old. It was unbelievable that she would die. Marie refused to accept it.

~*~

A few months later, Jackie called her and was crying. She had used up all her sick leave and all the sick leave her co-workers could donate to her, and now she wasn't able to work and had no money. She had an unemployed friend, Linda, who moved in with her and was helping to take care of her.

Jackie said," I called my boss and asked him about getting food stamps and he said I wasn't eligible. He said they were only for clients and that Child Welfare workers couldn't get them."

Marie shook her head. "Oh Jackie, that is utterly ridiculous. Food stamps are for any citizen who doesn't have income. You are eligible. Put Linda on the extension and I'll tell her what to do."

Marie then explained what documents they would need, and in what order, to qualify for food stamps. Linda wrote it all down, and Marie directed, "Now, go in at 8 a.m. on Friday morning. That is the slowest time of the week and you'll get immediate attention."

On Friday afternoon, Linda called her to tell her they got their food stamps and she had already been to the store. "Thank you, Marie; it was easy because of you. It was funny—the worker asked me, suspiciously, 'who helped me?' I told her you did, and that Jackie was a state worker. She couldn't have been more helpful after that."

"That is the least I could do, and call me if you ever have any questions. I'll be easier to get ahold of than your worker."

By now, Jackie was too weak for visitors, and Marie became more depressed. She spent most of her time reading. Five months after Ted left, at seven forty-five on a Friday night, the phone rang. Marie knew right away it was Ted calling. Who else would call her on a Friday night?

She didn't want him to think she was home alone on a Friday night, so she waited a few minutes and sure enough, in fifteen minutes the phone rang again. Now Marie was certain it was him. When he was impatient to reach her, he called every fifteen minutes until she answered the phone.

She got up from bed where she was reading a book and straightened up the apartment. Next Marie took a shower and washed her hair, dried and fixed it, and put on make-up. The whole time she was doing this, the telephone rang every fifteen minutes. She was excited that he was calling her, though she didn't know if he was in town or not. Finally, the suspense got to her and she picked up the phone at eleven-thirty. She hadn't planned what she would say.

"Hey," Ted said, "Can I come home?"

Marie hesitated for about fifteen seconds; she knew she should tell him she was busy, and someone was in the apartment. He calls her out of the blue on a Friday night after five months of no contact and expects her to be free?

However, he melted her heart when he asked if he could come home, and she said, “Sure.”

He was there in ten minutes and they had quite a reunion. She was in his arms at the door and in the bed a few seconds later. Their clothes came off in a blizzard. Again, the sex was wonderful and they hadn’t forgotten anything. The two of them were completely compatible in bed and each knew what would pleasure the other.

Afterwards he asked, “Can I stay with you until I get an apartment?” And again, she said, “Sure.”

Within a week, they were back in their usual routine. He stayed out late and brought home food; she didn’t ask any questions. Marie didn’t know if he was looking for a job or if he was waiting for another out-of-town assignment. She just decided to wait and see what happened.

One Saturday night, Linda, the friend who was staying with Jackie, called to say that Jackie wanted to see her. Marie was surprised when Linda told her that Jackie didn’t expect to live for another week. Marie completely banished the thought of Jackie’s death and was not ready to face it, but she went to her house that night.

Marie was surprised at how she looked. Jackie had lost about fifty pounds and her eyes tracked separately. She sounded the same, and refused to wallow in sadness or regret. Her family was coming next week, so this was Marie’s evening with her.

Marie saw an Easter lily on the coffee table. “Jackie, I can’t believe it. Did someone actually send you that?”

“God, it is so tasteless. I suppose they want me to lie on the couch with the lily on my chest until I die.”

We laughed despite ourselves.

“You know what? I don’t have to deal with the trauma of turning forty. There was a time when I thought that would bother me, but I can forget about it. I’ll never see forty.” She stood up and turned around slowly, “See, I always wanted to weigh one-twenty and look at me now.”

Linda and Marie laughed because it was obvious that she would not tolerate sadness. Jackie knew Marie didn’t like to go to funerals. “I know you’ll find something better to do than to go to my funeral. I know you—but you better be there.”

“Yes, Jackie, I will come to your funeral come hell or high water. I wouldn’t miss it.”

Turning serious, Jackie said, “I want you to promise me that my casket will be closed. “I don’t want people to see me like this. I don’t mind you seeing me, but not anyone else.’

Marie would not have any control over her funeral, but she promised, “Jackie, I swear you will have a closed casket. I will make certain of that.”

Marie cast a glance at Linda, who nodded slightly. After a couple of hours, after Jackie tired, Marie hugged her one last time, and then stumbled outside to the lawn to weep in the dark. Linda followed her out, not to comfort her, but because she couldn’t hold back the tears any longer.

Jackie died early Wednesday morning, with her mother and sister at her side. Marie knew she would never have a friend as close to her again. Her funeral was to be Friday. Marie asked her big boss about the mandatory training she had on the job Friday, who said,

“I know you have to go to training on the day you are assigned and there are no exceptions, but my old supervisor at Child Welfare has died and I need to go to her funeral.”

“That’s too bad, but your current job is the most important. You have to go to your training.”

Marie was upset that she might miss Jackie’s funeral, especially after promising her she would be there, but she thought she could figure something out.

On Thursday evening, Ted came home early. Out of a clear blue sky, he said, "Let's start acting like adults and get an apartment together."

Marie was stunned and speechless and hardly knew what to think. This was completely out of left field. But she was still deeply grieving for Jackie and wondering how she was going to get to the funeral the next day. They would have to find another apartment if they moved in together and there was her lease to work out. She was not capable of thinking of it all right then.

"Okay," she said, and left the details until later. Not everything had to be decided right this moment.

On Friday morning, Ted told her he had left some of his things in Indianapolis—the last place he worked—and that he had to go back and pick them up. He said, "I'll be back on Monday."

Marie asked, out of an abundance of experience, "Do you mean next Monday? The one after tomorrow and Sunday?"

Ted said, "Yes," and they said good-bye as Marie hurried off to work.

At her training session, almost in tears, she said to the trainer, "I want to take off this afternoon to go to Jackie's funeral but I was told by the program director that was impossible. I don't see how I can miss that funeral."

The trainer, with tears welling up in her eyes said. "I don't have the authority to let you off, but I want to go to the funeral, too."

Several others chimed in. So the trainer asked, "Do the rest of you mind if we skip breaks and end training early this afternoon?"

The others agreed, and they did that.

When Marie got to the church, it was standing room only. She immediately and thankfully noted that the casket was closed. The church was packed and she saw all the people she had worked with when Jackie was her supervisor eleven years before.

She also went to the house afterward. There, Linda told her, "Tina showed up the last night while I was at the store. She attacked Jackie and took her pain medication. Jackie had to die without it. And I wish you could have seen her family fighting over her stuff. It was really sickening."

The whole thing was awful, but at least Marie had something to look forward to when Ted came back.

Chapter Fifteen

Marie went to work Monday morning with Jackie's funeral and a long, hard weekend behind her. Of course, she grieved for Jackie, but she knew when she went home tonight Ted would be there. Together they would start a new life. She was amazed this had happened. She never really believed Ted wanted to live with her or even acknowledge her as his girlfriend. Therefore, despite her sorrow, she looked forward to getting home Monday night.

Somehow, she wasn't surprised that he wasn't home when she got there. Well, he was probably out drinking or maybe he hadn't made it back to town yet. His being late was no reason for her to go into a panic. He wasn't home by the time she went to bed or when she left for work in the morning.

Tuesday she drove to work on a lovely day, but hardly noticed the weather. She was feeling a bit ambivalent. When she got to work, she went to Bobbie's office to tell her, "Ted hasn't come back yet, but I am trying to be calm about it. There are lots of reasons why he wouldn't be back yet. I managed to get to Jackie's funeral Friday, but it was a near thing. It's hard to believe that she was my supervisor in the Child Welfare Department, but Food Stamps wouldn't let me off for her funeral. I guess it's typical."

Bobbie agreed, "Yes, it is a shame that the Department doesn't care about its employees. I'm glad you made it to the funeral; and I'm glad you aren't making a big deal of Ted being late coming back. He'll show up.

Marie worked all day, hardly even thinking of Ted. But on her way home, she wondered if he would be there when she got there. He wasn't, and he didn't call. She stayed up late for him, but he didn't show.

The next day she was distracted at work, thinking of whether or not he would come home that day. It was Wednesday, and he promised to be back on Monday. She told Bobbie, "Whatever story he tells me, it'll be good."

They both laughed, and she went home. She stopped by the mailbox, as she always did on the way to her apartment; it was right outside her front door. This afternoon there was a letter with familiar handwriting. Marie's heart dropped and she swayed with dizziness. It was the first time Ted wrote her and she knew it wouldn't be good news.

When she opened the envelope in her living room, a check fell out. It was made out to her, for three hundred dollars. The note said, "Here is the money I owe you. I'll see you later. Don't try to contact me. Ted"

Marie was devastated. She knew he would not be paying her the money he owed unless he didn't intend to see her again. She checked the note again. It was postmarked in Oklahoma City, no return address. Marie cried, and then she lit a joint to try to kill the pain.

It was a suddcn cnd to their relationship that lasted just a few months short of ten years, but he always showed up again before. And there was that suggestion that they move in together last week. Did he scare himself by almost making a commitment? In her heart, she refused to give up on ever seeing him again. However, she thought it would be weeks or maybe months or years before she did.

Marie didn't miss a day of work, but there wasn't a day that she didn't weep on the way home from work—she would hold the tears back all day until she got in the car to go home, then would start to cry. She steeled herself for a long wait before

Ted changed his mind, and started to slide back into depression.

Bobbie told her, “You are better off without him. Now maybe you can find someone who will treat you right.”

Marie heard that from every friend she had ever told about Ted. There was no Jackie to confide in and no one understood. Her family was particularly happy that Ted was gone. It was true that her mother was sympathetic because she knew it hurt to lose someone you cared about so much. Her father said, “I am glad that SOB is gone. I never liked the way he treated you.”

Even Shirley said, “You are better off without him.”

The funny thing was she had no desire to date anyone; all she wanted to do was to wait for Ted to come home. For months, on Saturday mornings at two, she would wake up and wait for the phone to ring. It never did. Marie stayed home every evening, waiting for the phone. Last time she waited for five months, and he called. If she waited long enough this time, he would call again.

Many times, she felt like ending it all, and once had a vision of herself with a butcher knife stuck halfway through her throat. It was vivid, almost like a hallucination. She wondered if she was supposed to go to the kitchen and get her biggest knife and saw through her neck, but whenever she thought of suicide, even this time, even though she was serious about it, she held herself back with the thought that Ted might return. Then she would be happy and killing herself would have been a mistake.

Marie started to lose more weight as she slid back into depression. Her clothes looked bigger and bigger. She didn’t try to buy any new ones; she just wore them as they were. She wasn’t feeling well and finally she went to a doctor. She told him,

"I haven't been feeling well. I don't sleep at all well, and I have been losing weight. My knee, which I have not injured, has begun to hurt me constantly and I don't know why."

The doctor, a rheumatologist, examined her carefully and said, "Your knee hurts, and I believe that. However, you have a nervous type of pain, which cannot be helped by painkillers. All I can tell you to do is to stop worrying so much and to eat an egg a day to improve your nutrition."

Marie realized her pain was related to her depression and there was nothing to be done for it. Trying to follow the doctor's orders, she started stopping at a 24-hour café every morning on the way to work for an egg, hash browns, toast, and coffee. In a corner, they had a doctor's scale, and Marie gasped aloud when it registered only ninety-nine pounds. A woman there asked what was wrong, and Marie said, "only ninety-nine pounds!"

The woman said, "That's too skinny. You had better start eating more."

It seemed to her that she was eating enough, but she was not gaining any weight. At five feet, five inches, that was much thinner than she wanted to be, but she seemed to have no control over it.

She thought about getting some counseling, and remembered the time she tried counseling the year before, when the psychologist told her just to get over her depression. That was so frustrating she didn't want to go through it again. If she knew how to get over it, she would. She felt about an inch tall, and questioned herself constantly as to why she hadn't been good enough for Ted. She certainly tried to make him happy, but nothing she did was right.

At work, the frustrations of the job started to get to her. She didn't take it out on the clients, but on her fellow workers. Bobbie told her, "You messed up on this computer form and they sent it back." Marie replied, looking at the form, "Oh no, this form is correct. I didn't make a mistake on it!" Bobbie leaned over her shoulder and pointed out her error. "By cracky goddamn! I can't believe I made that mistake!" Marie exclaimed.

She punched a filing cabinet and yelled at another worker when she came in to work and had forgotten it was her duty day. "I had my day all planned and knew just what work I was going to do and now you tell me I have the duty and won't be able to do what I had planned!" Marie was livid.

Bobbie understood and put up with her moods at this time, but the other workers got impatient with her. She wasn't easy to work with and not much fun to be around.

A year went by, and Marie hadn't heard a word from Ted. She wrote him a couple of letters and sent them to him at his friend's houses, but they came back to her "No such addressee." Marie knew it would be a long time before she heard from him, so she just dug in for the long haul.

One night when she got home from work, she found Neko lying on her side on the bed, panting. She looked awful. Marie knew Neko was quite ill when she didn't respond to her. She called her regular vet to make sure that someone would wait for her and bundled Neko into the car and rushed to the vet's office. On the way to the office, Nek screamed as she usually did when taken for a ride in the car, so Marie thought that maybe she would be okay.

When they arrived, the vet simply took Neko and told Marie to go home. Marie had a bad feeling and went to one of her friend's home who was also a cat person. She drank a little and cried a lot.

The next morning she called the vet's office. When the vet got on the phone, he said, "I'm sorry, but Neko died just as I put her on the table last night. Her kidneys have completely failed her. I tried to call you last night but couldn't reach you."

Marie began crying. "Thank you for all you have done for her over the years—especially all the times you stitched her up after her fights. Now I'm going to ask you to help me find another cat."

"I'll be happy to—I know you are a good cat mother."

Marie hung up. She felt she had lost everyone who ever loved her. She knew that was an exaggeration, but she would miss Neko. She had been her companion for thirteen years.

Chapter Sixteen

Marie had just got to work and sat at her battered wooden desk sipping her first cup of coffee from the office coffee pot, thinking about getting ready for her first client. The fluorescent light overhead flickered and hummed. A wave of sadness quaked inside her and she took a big gulp of coffee trying to wash it away. She reached for the middle drawer, where she kept her personal stuff, and pulled out a pocket mirror to check how puffy her eyes were. The light slanted through her window where dirty stains were left from the time someone lobbed a tomato at it five year ago; no one had ever bothered to clean it. Next to the window, the paint was peeling off the wall. Why am I still here, she asked herself. Bobbie's head popped in the door.

"We are having an emergency meeting with a guy from state office in half an hour, so get ready. It's going to be bad."

Marie rested her forehead in her hand and sighed. She got up, got more coffee from the communal coffee pot, and wondered if they would ever get good news.

The meeting started with the usual fake bonhomie, then the man, Mr. Briggs, bald and mustachioed, cut right to the chase and explained that there was a problem. Marie held her breath. She gulped a mouthful of coffee next to brace herself. "We took the lowest bid on software for Food Stamps uses," he said, "and it turned out to be incompatible with our hardware. Until we can work the problem out, food stamps will be issued manually, without a computer. You workers need to do all the work that the computer did plus your regular work."

Marie's head reeled. Somebody asked, "How can we do that?"

"Oh," Mr. Briggs said, "You will be allowed to use whatever method works best for you. Your supervisors will help you. Well, good luck with it. I'm sure that you all will handle it well."

Everyone was already scheduled with clients, so there were only a few moments to react. Marie felt sick, and it didn't help her mood at all when Ruby leaned over to comment, "You know someone took a bribe to choose that particular software." They all complained in an uproar to Bobbie, who wasn't any happier, but she listened for a little while, and then redirected them to think about their appointments.

She didn't think she would get through the day but made it with an upset stomach and indigestion from all the coffee she drank. Between appointments, what little time she had, she doodled as she tried to plan ways to manage her caseload. Let's see, I could—no, that wouldn't work, or maybe I could, no... After she got home that night, she sat in bed with a notebook and realized it had only been a few years that computers had been used. There had to be a way to do paperwork without them. She smoked a pack while she figured it out.

Marie went to the office the next day with a strong step. It was her duty day, so she didn't have appointments. In between drop-in clients, she put into effect the plan she made the night before by taking index cards and making up a tickler file with the client's name and certification date. With this, she thought, I can keep track of those who need appointments and who is already certified and needs stamps each month. It will be a pain, but I just need to keep these updated and filed. The next thing will have to be filling out the forms for everyone who is certified every month and then dumping them on the poor clerk who was going to type and mail the stamps each month. She knew it would work, as long as she didn't get distracted.

Marie sighed. She asked Bobbie, "How am I going to keep up with all this paperwork without messing up and forgetting to get stamps to someone who was already certified? You know there are federal government time mandates I have to meet and I am expected to meet all the requirements. These rules don't say, 'Unless your state welfare office screws up and you don't have a computer.' "

Bobbie said, "I know it's scary, but I am not worried about you—you always get your work done. I have six others to worry about."

Marie sat in her office and looked around, discouraged. There was a pile of cases under her feet, and one sitting on the bookcase, and one in the chair. Hey, it works for me, but what happens if I get sick? To someone else it's a mess, not a system.

At each interview, Marie said, "Our computer is messed up so I have to get your Stamps to you by hand. Now don't worry," she'd say, taking a drag on her cigarette, "I can do it. Now, don't call me if you don't get your stamps right away, but do call me if you don't get them in a reasonable time."

Most of her clients left happy, and one of them answered, "I'm not worried. So far, you've been faster than the computer."

Marie was drinking more coffee and smoking more. One day another worker pointed out an error she made and she yelled, "What business is it of yours?" The worker, cringing, said, "I was only trying to help, but don't worry, it won't happen again."

Marie wanted to apologize, but the words stuck in her throat. She asked Bobbie, "Why did I do all that work to get a Masters' Degree if all I was ever going to do was interview people for Food Stamps?"

It was scary, so she started checking the job boards for the department. She wouldn't apply for anything in state office, because it was well-known that you had to sleep with someone in personnel to get a job there and she didn't want a job that bad. God, she thought, I'd rather starve.

However, there were jobs she could fill as worker II, III, or supervisor. She filled out application after application and psyched herself up for interviews. She would cry quietly in her office when they came to nothing, square her shoulders, and get back to work.

Marie wondered, and she didn't know, if her reputation for being difficult had preceded her, or if there was a lot of affirmative action going on. It seemed like it was both. She had no control and many times, rather than be sad, she would get mad and pound her desk.

One day Marie had been turned down for two jobs she had real hopes for. The dingy office, the (small number of fraudulent) clients, the absolutely amazing ignorance of her colleagues, the frustration of doing the same thing over and over for the rest of her life, had her crying, slinging files around her office, and showing off her considerable repertoire of curse words.

Suddenly Bobbie stuck her head in the door. She said, in a cool tone, "Marie, get a cup of coffee and come to my office, I need to talk with you."

Marie knew it couldn't be good. She was doing a good job, keeping up with her cases, but somehow she didn't think that Bobbie had picked that moment to tell her that. She went to the coffee pot, filled up her mug, checked her supply of cigarettes, and marched off to Bobbie's office.

Bobbie's office was just as dingy as everyone else's. It was just a little larger. Bobbie shut the door and lit a cigarette, which Marie copied. Bobbie wanted to talk about Marie's mood and her frustrations with the job. She said, "I know you have done the best you could under the circumstances, but I can't have you acting the way you are in the office. There is a belief that state workers can't be fired, but you know that isn't true."

Marie knew that Bobbie had earned her supervisory position by ridding the department of a problem employee by careful documentation and tireless counseling as a Worker II.

"I don't want to have to go through all that with you. It will ruin our friendship and I don't want to do that, plus it is a tremendous amount of work. You and I both know you are not happy here. You've worked this job too long. I'll let you give two weeks' notice and we'll tell people you are resigning because you found a better job.

Marie thought about it and knew she didn't have a choice. She felt more relief than anger or dismay. The thought of not having to deal with the stress of the job was enough to make her feel better immediately. She asked, "Could I have a little time to look for a job before I give notice? I have worked here for seven years, as you said."

"Yes, you can have that. You have done a good job here and have always showed up for work and tried to do a good job. Just let me know how your job search is going."

Marie started the next day, checking the ads in the paper. She was surprised to see that a private school was advertising for a full-time social studies teacher. That sounded really good, so she called and got an appointment for an interview.

She had to mesh the interview into her Food Stamp schedule, but finally worked it out. She was excited at the thought of teaching. She had a teacher's certificate in social studies, but had never used it except part time in junior colleges.

The school was way out by Quail Springs Mall. It was located in a new, modern building that didn't look much like a school. It looked more like a strip mall than a school. It was named the "Cooper School" and had only a few students, maybe seventy-five. It was an alternative school for students, who, for various reasons, could not make it or were not happy with public schools.

Marie talked with the owners of the school, a married couple, Lloyd and Dimity John. Marie was so nervous she could hardly speak. Lloyd was a huge blond man and Dimity was a tiny, stylish woman with frosted hair. Soon Marie found that their philosophy of educating teenagers was close to her own.

Lloyd said, "The students learn at their own pace as we teach them one at a time."

"Oh, so it will be like tutoring; I'll only have one student at a time in the class?"

"Yes, that's right. Some students need to learn more slowly, and some need to have the material enriched. Because our students often come from emotionally deprived homes, they are encouraged to ask any questions they want. Our teachers are expected to answer any question they do ask, no matter what the subject."

"Okay, I understand," Marie said.

"And another thing—they call their teachers by their first names. We encourage informality and closeness between teacher and student."

"I agree with the way your teaching philosophy but I've never been called by my first name by students. I guess I can get used to it. I love working with teenagers, though I know they can be difficult at times."

"Well, until you've worked in a school like this, you probably don't know how difficult they can be; but there are also many rewards when the students respond to you. I think you will fit in well here."

The only problem was the salary. It almost, but did not completely, pay her expenses. She would come up a little short each month. However, Marie really needed a job and she could squeak by until she found a better job if she took her retirement money from the state. She happily signed on with the school, and the Johnsons seemed pleased to get her, too.

Marie was so relieved to have a job and to think that she would not have to face clients all day, every day, anymore. She would not have to try to do her job and the computer's, too. She went back to the office and told Bobbie, "I've found a teaching job that will start in August."

"That's great, Marie, stay on until it is convenient for you to leave, then give me notice and we'll tell everyone about your new job and give you a going-away party. No one will ever need to know that I asked you to resign and you won't have to put it on your résumé."

Leaving the frustrating Food Stamp job was going to take a lot of pressure off Marie. She hoped it would ease her depression and give her interesting things to think about, rather than feeling sorry for herself all the time and thinking about Ted.

Chapter Seventeen

Marie was "on vacation." She resigned from her Food Stamps job two weeks before the teaching job started. Lying in her bed, reading, taking it easy, she suddenly felt as if someone hit her in the middle of her back with a sledgehammer. She wondered how she could be in such serious pain.

She walked carefully, stooped over, to the table where she kept the Yellow Pages. Lighting up a cigarette, she paged through the ads, finding a doctor who specialized in back pain and punched in the numbers. "Hey, I just suddenly have this awful pain. Do you think you could see me today?"

The clerk asked, "Are you a new patient?" and Marie sighed. "Yes, I am a new patient, I just suddenly had this back pain and I don't know why." "Okay," the clerk answered. "The doctor can see you at two."

She wondered how soon this could be cleared up. She slipped into the most comfortable, easiest clothes she could find, stepping into them carefully, as if they were a trap.

Marie painfully settled into the driver's seat of her car, and found that she could not turn her head without a sharp stab of pain. Gingerly, she pressed the accelerator and carefully drove, watching the lights compulsively; afraid one would change too fast for her to swing her foot to the brake. It would be awful to rear-end someone.

At the doctor's office, she had to lie on the floor until the doctor could see her. She could not tolerate sitting in a chair, leaning against the back of the chair put too much pressure on her back. She felt a little foolish, but the pain was such that she just stared at the ceiling and ignored the other patients. First, the nurse had her stand for an X-ray. Then the doctor saw her. Marie said, "I'm really scared I have done some damage. It hurts so bad."

The doctor was quite open with her. "Are you crazy?" he asked.

Marie nodded her head, agreeing that she wasn't quite right. "There is nothing wrong with you. Your body played a trick on you. You were so upset about something that your back muscles spasmed and pinched your spine." She looked at him in shock, but with some relief that there was no physical damage.

"Well, if I am okay, why does it hurt so much?" Marie asked him, irritably.

The doctor explained that she just needed muscle relaxers and rest. Then he asked, "Are you doing something right now that is causing you stress?"

"Only starting a new job, but I wanted to change jobs. Marie shook her head. "Guess I scared myself."

"Just stay in bed a couple of days and take the muscle relaxers. You'll be fine."

Marie felt stupid and got out of the office as fast as her condition would let her, which meant she hobbled out. Relief was her main emotion; she found it hard to believe that one could worry oneself into such a state.

She lay in bed anxious but resting, while she thought about her new job. Thumbing through her college syllabi, she smoked and twirled her hair around her finger. Marie would be teaching American history, world history, and government to about ten students. The thought of this made her stomach flip-flop, so she dug out some college notes and made outlines, trying to get ahead of the game. As she looked them over, she realized what a big job she had taken on: five classes on

Monday and Wednesday and five classes to different students on Tuesday and Thursday. Classes did not meet on Friday, so that was her time to prepare.

On her first day, she drove to work, impatiently negotiating the construction zones.

She had tried several routes to the job, and all of the streets going north were torn up. She thought this one would be the best, but it still made her crazy and she cursed under her breath at the other drivers. She calmed down after arriving at school and having her first cup of coffee.

She met her students one by one, as they came to class. Arturo, her first on Monday morning, was skinny and had long, dark, unkempt hair. He struck her as detached and she was told he was a drug abuser. He had signed a contract with the school that he would come to school every day, he would be on time, and he would not be high at school.

James, her second student, looked to her to be a friendly, pleasant small boy in her world history class. Unfortunately, Marie realized on the first day that either his hobby was driving her crazy, or he was truly horribly confused. He stated, when she opened with some remarks about the Middle Ages, that "Martin Luther and Martin Luther King, Jr. were the same people, weren't they?" When she tried to explain, "No, they weren't—Martin Luther was a religious dissenter in the Middle Ages and Martin Luther King was a contemporary Civil Rights leader, he just looked at her with a goofy grin. She realized he said that just to annoy her.

A blond, gangly girl, Lydia, an American history student, was rambunctious and thought she was an adult. One of the tenets of the school was that teachers would answer any question the student asked, so Marie found herself answering "How old were you when you got your first apartment and car?" Lydia's face fell when Marie said, "I got my first apartment when I was twenty-one and my first car at twenty-five." She was trying to get ammunition to get her parents to let her move out of the house at seventeen. Marie's answers were obviously not the ones the child was looking for. Marie knew what she wanted and smiled to herself as she answered.

The next student, Dora, was fourteen years old, a sweet little girl with dark hair and big brown eyes. Dora asked her, "How do you make hard-boiled eggs?" Marie told her, and was surprised by her answer when she asked her why she wanted to know.

"My stepmother," Dora said, "orders in fried chicken one week and pizza for the next week that's all we ever have to eat. Sometimes I feel like eating something else."

Last was Angela, tall, self-possessed, with black hair and perfect posture, so intelligent she simply didn't have the patience to sit in a regular classroom. She was from a prominent Hispanic family who owned a string of restaurants called the "Gallery" in town. Marie sensed that Angela was more intelligent than she was, but it was easy to accelerate the subject for her because Marie knew much more on the subject than she did. Angela kept Marie on her toes. It was fun to teach her and they could converse on almost an adult level.

Unfortunately, after a few weeks, Arturo was cut from the school. He came in late too many times, and was high on drugs when he did attend. Marie breathed a sigh of relief when she found out he wouldn't be back. He was a trial to teach, since he didn't pay attention and always wanted to go off on tangents. At the same time, she was upset that he wasn't getting an education. The Cooper School was probably his last chance.

James never let up on her. He refused to learn anything she tried to teach him. He was the student who gave her the most trouble and try as she might, she never got through to him. She talked with the boss about him, but he didn't have any suggestions for sparking his interest. She dreaded his class time and made sure she smoked a cigarette before she tried to work with him.

She was preparing for class one night, it seemed like she was never caught up, when she answered the phone and was startled to be talking to the father of her students, Carolyn. He was a lawyer, and Marie wondered what kind of trouble she was in this time. She drew in her breath sharply, but he just said, "I wanted to tell you Carolyn is enjoying and learning history for the first time in her life. I don't know what you are doing, but she is asking me questions about history and talking to me about it. I have always thought that history is important and it is a joy to see my child interested. I just wanted to tell you how grateful I am."

"Carolyn seems interested in class and I'm glad that I have been able to inspire her. I love history, too and I guess I have communicated that to her," said Marie. Carolyn's response made it worth all the work to Marie.

Dora came to class one Monday seemingly calm and collected, but she quietly asked, "What is an abortion like?"

Marie's heart petrified. No, she thought, Dora's only fourteen. Marie explained what an abortion was, and then asked, "Dora, are you going to have one?"

Dora answered, matter of factly, "My father, stepmother and mother have scheduled one for me but haven't told me what it was like or even if it will hurt."

Marie drew in her breath and said, "Yes, it will hurt some but it won't be more than you can handle." Marie was able to keep from crying because she didn't want to upset Dora. That was the first time the term "poor little rich girl" popped into Marie's head.

During one class, Angela asked her "Isn't it okay for a person to have all the children she wants as long as she can support them?" Marie countered, judiciously, since Angela came from a big family, by reminding her that "the earth has limited resources, and that should be taken into consideration, but that is a decision each person must make." She could tell that Angela did not agree.

Chapter Eighteen

On Halloween, one of the students threw a party. Marie put on red and white footed pajamas and had her neighbor, Sharon, make her up as a clown. Sharon did a great job; looking in the mirror Marie hardly recognized herself. She had red cheeks, big black eyebrows, huge red lips, a red ball for a nose, and a red clown wig.

When she got to the party, feeling somewhat ridiculous, only some of her students recognized her. One of them started to introduce her to his parent, then said, "This is kind of embarrassing, but meet Marie, my history teacher." They all laughed.

Marie enjoyed the teaching and the interaction with the students, but she realized regretfully, she could pull it off for only one year. She had really learned to love the place and the people. It simply didn't pay her enough to continue working there.

She was still hung up on Ted, but by now, after almost two years since he left, she had pretty much given up on his returning. Incredibly, Marie still regularly woke up at 2 a.m., expectantly waiting for the phone to ring.

She had not gained any weight and her mood had not improved as much as she had hoped it would. She hadn't made any close friends with the other teachers, but she had pleasant relationships with some of them. One afternoon after classes an English teacher, Rose, came into her room and said, "My husband and I are having trouble paying our electric bill this month; you know how hot it's been. Could you lend us two hundred and fifty dollars just until payday?"

Marie was startled that someone she didn't know well would ask for a loan. However, she had loaned money to people for years, and they had always paid her back. She also just didn't know how to say, "No." She was embarrassed and just wanted to get out of the situation. The thought hit her, will it hurt me here if I don't loan her the money? She really didn't want to do it, but Marie wrote them a check and tried not to worry about it.

When payday came, the teacher told her it would be a couple more weeks. This went on for a month or two, until Marie realized that she wasn't going to get her money back. She confronted the English teacher, Rose, who said, "No, we aren't going to pay the money back. We just don't have it."

"Why did you borrow it from me in the first place?"

"We thought we could pull it off but we couldn't, sorry."

Marie couldn't believe she was so casual about basically just taking money from her. She chastised herself for lending money to someone she hardly knew, and told herself she would learn from it. Marie felt so stupid.

Marie had continued her habit of eating breakfast at the café each morning. It didn't cost much and was easier than cooking for herself—and the doctor had emphasized the nutrition she needed.

After several months, she struck up an acquaintance with a good-looking, pleasant man named Patrick who was in the café every day at the same time she was. He had black, curly hair, blue eyes and a big smile. Patrick only had nice things to say about anyone, and she thought she could like him.

They spoke about the weather or the headlines for a while, and then began to get more personal. When she asked Patrick what he did, he said, "I'm the district supervisor for the distribution of the morning newspaper. I have several people who report to me, but I don't actually throw the papers unless someone is sick or can't get to work for some reason."

They inevitably started an intimate relationship within the month and one time he commented that, unlike most women, "You don't wear any diamonds." Marie told him she had never been married, so never had a man given her a diamond.

The next time she saw him, he gave her a tiny diamond necklace, "This will make sure you have a diamond, as you should have."

Marie said, "Thank you, that is so kind," but laughed to herself because the diamond was so small you could barely see it with the naked eye. She said to herself, just what I need to feel wanted, a diamond you have to look at through a microscope.

"Patrick," she told him, I have taken nine thousand dollars in retirement funds from my welfare job, and I am saving it to live on until I could get a better-paying job. I love teaching like this, and I would like to keep doing it, but I can't afford it."

Patrick exclaimed, "I have a great idea. I have just started a small business and if you invest in it, I will give you a 12% interest rate. It will help me with capital and you'll get a good return for your money."

"This money is precious to me. I need it to live on until I can find a job that completely supports me. I don't think so."

"No," said Patrick, "nothing can go wrong. This is a surefire deal. You'll be helping me out by supplying me with money up front, and as I make money, I will be able to pay you back with a good interest rate. We'll put in in writing."

Marie hated to say "no" to him and when he said he would put the conditions in writing she agreed. After all, a man who she was sleeping with wouldn't cheat her, would he? That night he brought the agreement to her house and they both signed it. Patrick agreed to borrow $1,500 and to pay it back, with 12% interest, in a month.

Marie went to the bank the next day and withdrew they money from her savings account. She was still hesitant about the whole thing and again, when Patrick came to pick up the money, reminded him of how much she counted on him. She really felt bad about this whole thing, but would he stop liking her if she wouldn't give him the money?

"Patrick, I've got to have this money back. This is not extra money I have. It is money I need to live on until I find another job."

"Oh, I know. There is no problem. You'll have it back, with interest, in no time."

Chapter Nineteen

Marie couldn't wait to blow her money on one thing she always wanted. When Neko died, she promised herself a pair of pedigreed cats. Tearfully, she asked the vet, "Do you know any breeders of pedigreed cats who also raise them well?

He said, "I know one who raises Burmese cats and treats them like family."

Marie called the number he gave her and the breeder, Ms. Anderson said, "Do you want show quality or just a kitten?"

Marie answered, "It doesn't matter to me. I don't intend to show them, though."

Ms. Anderson said, "Well, I have two kittens ready to go right now; one is a show-quality female and the other is not show-quality, but he is a special little male."

"How much do you want for them?'

"Since they are not both show-quality, I'm asking only $350 for the pair. I would be especially happy if you kept them together."

"When can I come over and see them?"

"How about this afternoon?"

Marie said, "Great." She felt like it had already been too long since there was a cat in the house.

When she arrived, it was a perfectly kept duplex, half for Ms. Anderson and her son, the other half for the cats. It was an efficient way to run a cat-breeding business and impressed

Marie with its cleanliness and how pleasant it was. Ms. Anderson brought the kittens out in a little basket. "Oh," Marie exclaimed, "they are gorgeous." Her heart leapt when she saw them.

They had chartreuse eyes peering out of deep, dark brown fur. Each hair in their coats was tipped with silver, so they shone. Despite being pedigreed, fancy and expensive, they acted like any other kittens, with the male rolling over immediately for Marie to rub his tummy. She played with them, laughed at them and then she pulled out her checkbook. Knowing she would love them at first sight, she had brought along her cat carrier.

She named the male Phideaux.

The breeder's son said, "You see how small he is. He was the runt of the litter and I babied him. Once he was old enough to pick up, I carried him everywhere on my shoulder. He is definitely spoiled rotten, but he also has a preference for men."

Because of this, Phideaux was always getting himself into to trouble. He followed men into apartments and was locked in. Once he followed a construction crew into their workshop and he got locked in.

Marie knew exactly where he was and she went to the foreman and asked him, "Please, will you go back to the workshop and let my cat out?

He laughed at her, "Lady, your cat is just out tom-catting around. He's not in our workshop."

She was not surprised when Phideaux showed up the next morning at 8 a.m.

He disappeared regularly during the day and Marie finally discovered that one of her neighbors, who worked the night shift, left his balcony door open while he slept. Phideaux would creep into his bedroom and sleep with him. If Marie missed him, she learned to call that neighbor's wife and ask, "Is Phideaux in bed with your husband?"

Sharon would check and come back to say, "Yes, he is—do you want me to send him home or can he stay for a while?"

Marie said, "He can stay until Travis wakes up, but then send him home." At least she knew where he was.

Marie named her little female cat Peave. She was a drama queen who bonded immediately with Marie. At the end of Peave's first week, Marie came home from work to find her limping. She rushed her to the vet, knowing there would be emergency fee. The vet pronounced the tiny, limping kitten to be "the most pitiful sight I have ever seen."

The vet x-rayed the leg, felt the bone and could find nothing wrong. "Just take her home and observe her, and bring her back if she doesn't improve."

When Marie got her home, still so worried she couldn't think of eating dinner, Peave leapt out of her arms and ran around the apartment with no sign of a limp. She was like that the rest of her life; if Peave didn't feel well, she put on such a show that she had to go to the vet, where they called her "Sarah Barnhardt."

She also was a cuddly cat, and if Marie left home to go anywhere but work, Peave sat patiently at the entrance to the complex, waiting for her to come home. The cats lifted Marie's spirits and gave her something to love and to think about. Every time she sat down, she had a squirming pile of love in her lap and she wasn't so lonely anymore.

Patrick came over regularly in the morning, playing with the kittens and telling her, "Hey, the new business is doing great."

After the month was up, Marie said, "I'd like to have my money back now."

Patrick replied, "it'll be another week before I'm in a position to get it to you."

Then, suddenly Patrick didn't come around anymore. And since he was married, Marie had never learned his address or phone number. She knew how to reach him at work, but when she called him, the clerk said, “He isn’t in this afternoon.” Marie knew she had been taken, again.

She took their agreement to a lawyer, who said, “Your interest rate is usurious, therefore it is not a legal contract and you can’t do anything.” Years later, when she asked another lawyer, he said, “Since he suggested the interest rate, the whole thing is fraudulent and it is enforceable as fraud.”

By that time, Marie had lost total track of him and really didn’t want to pursue a claim for $1,500. It was embarrassing.

Marie asked herself, how could I have been so stupid? I gave away money to two people I don’t know well, and it was money I couldn’t afford to lose. She got more depressed and felt worse about herself. Marie began to wonder if living in the City was her problem. The happiest time of her life was when she went to Oklahoma University and lived in Norman. Things were simpler and she wasn’t always having all these problems.

What I need to do, she told herself, is to move back to Norman, find a job, and settle into a quieter lifestyle. She remembered that David, a guy she dated in college, still lived in Norman. She anxiously started to dial long distance information, then hesitated, and finally worked up the nerve to ask for his number.

When it was time to call him, she started to dial the number, then stopped, then finally finished it. The phone rang and someone answered. Marie said, tremulously, “David?”

He answered, “Yes.”

“David, it’s Marie. You know, from before you went in the Navy.”

“Oh my god!” he said, “It’s been so long! What, fifteen years?”

Marie and he hadn’t talked since that time.

On the phone, she said, “Yes it’s been a long time. “How have you been?”

David answered, "I've been fine, doing great. Why are you calling?"

"David, I am thinking about moving to Norman and I wonder what you think about that. I was hoping to get a job on campus." Marie was so depressed she had stopped watching TV or reading the newspapers. She really had no idea that the country was in the middle of a severe recession.

David answered, "I don't think that is a good idea. There is a hiring freeze on campus and not many jobs in Norman. I don't think it would work."

"I'd still like to come and check it out. Could I come down there and spend a Saturday with you and look around?"

"Sure," David said. "Come next weekend. I'll see you then." He said, "Come into town north of the campus, and drive down Main until you got to Sumac. My house is the third on the right." Marie carefully wrote it down.

"It's funny, David, but I will have trouble driving around Norman. When I went to school there I didn't have a car, so I only went places I could walk. Most of the town will be new territory to me."

David said, "You will also be astounded by how much it has grown."

On Saturday, Marie was excited and anxious. She started off for Norman, which was not a long drive, thinking that perhaps she had found someone to care about. Finding Dave's house with no problem, she noted that it was an average brick house; but there were no trees in the neighborhood, so it was somewhat bland.

Excited, she knocked on the door, and Dave answered. "Hey," he said, greeted her with a hug and a kiss.

"I didn't know if you would come since it is snowing."

"I don't usually drive in the snow, but I had promised to come and the interstate wasn't bad. It seems kind of late for snow."

"It does, but you know Oklahoma weather. After you warm up, I'd like to take you on a tour of the campus so you can see the changes.

"Oh, that sounds great."

"Let's get a burger first, then take drive around campus," David said.

When they got to the campus, David pointed, "See, there is the new social work building, and after you left they built a new history building."

"I'll bet that is nice; they probably have air-conditioning in the classrooms now." Marie wasn't too impressed until she saw the microbiology building—it was built the last year she attended school there, and then it looked raw and bare. Marie clapped her hands and exclaimed, "Look at the micro building. Now I really know I've been away. It is surrounded by all those beautiful trees."

Dave laughed too, "I hadn't even noticed the change."

When they returned home, they settled in the living room, which was plain and what Marie called male-decorated. David said, "Did you notice that no one around here has any trees?"

Marie said, "Yes, I did see that."

Dave explained "There are chemicals in the soil that preclude the growth of trees and I am disappointed in my yard. I would have liked to have had some nice elms."

Then he said, "I really don't think it would be a good idea for you to move here. As I told you, there is a job freeze on at the campus, and jobs are hard to find off-campus because students will do anything."

"Dave, you may be right but I really think that living in Norman will make me happy. I haven't made up my mind yet, but I am thinking about it."

"You should think some more."

"Okay, I will, I promise, David," Marie asked, after a pause, "why aren't you married?"

"You know why; and I don't want to talk about it."

David was engaged in his sophomore year, Marie remembered. He had finals to take and his girlfriend asked him to drive her to El Paso for Christmas because it was icy and she was afraid to go by herself. She had already taken her finals. David told her he had to stay in Norman and study; she would be fine. She started driving home, hit an icy patch, spun off the road and hit a tree. She was killed instantly. David didn't take the rest of his finals.

It was the Vietnam era, so, knowing he would lose his student deferment, he immediately enlisted in the Navy. However, since so many men had enlisted, he had to wait to be mustered in. Marie met David during the time he was in limbo. They had a light, several-months long relationship. David called her "Skinny" and he stayed with her whenever he was in town. While he was in basic, Marie sent him flirty postcards and a photo of herself in a bikini, which he showed around to the guys. Since he was older and had a "girlfriend," he was popular and was even elected "top recruit."

David came to see her after his basic training, but when Marie said, "I'll write to you and we can get together after you get out of the navy," David said, "No, I won't have you waiting for me. We'll say 'good-bye' now and that will be it." Marie could see he was still not over the death of his girlfriend, and her heart ached for him.

That evening David took her to her favorite hangout, a beer and pizza place, for dinner. There were students there, but also a sprinkling of guys Dave's age. Dave said, "I want to introduce you to a couple of my friends, Manny and Joe. Marie told them how she and Dave met back in college and they reminisced about their dating days. David told how he had a "metal Mustang" when he was waiting to enter the Navy, "and I stupidly sold it instead of keeping it until after I was discharged. It would be worth a mint now."

Manny and Joe laughed at this and Manny commented that "anyone who kept their Mustang would be rich now, because practically everyone has gotten rid of it."

Marie said, "I got lonesome for David while he was in basic. No one was allowed to call him except for emergencies, so I called and said his grandmother had died. David picked up the phone and said, "Skinny, what are you doing?"

They laughed all evening. After dinner, Marie said, "I'll head for home now; I want to get home early because of the snow."

'No, stay the night. You don't need to drive home in the dark and the snow."

Marie happily agreed. It was a little odd when, after they got to his house, he said, "I'm going to leave you alone while I go to the basketball game, but I only have one season ticket. Is that okay?"

Marie said, "I'll just read one of your books while you're gone. It'll be fine."

When he came home, they went to bed and had reminiscence sex. It was slow and easy but not passionate. Marie didn't mind; it felt warm and pleasant and she didn't think she would ever have sex like she did with Ted again. It was nice to be with someone she had a long connection with.

They woke up early in the morning, and then Marie said, "I really am eager to get home and see my cats." They ate a simple breakfast, and while they ate, David warmed her boots by the fire, and then helped her into them. Marie was so impressed; she told him, "I have never had my boots warmed up for me before. That was really nice"

Marie was so happy. As she drove home in the melting snow, she thought to herself that she had found a guy and she was going to move back to the town where she was happiest. Her life was going to turn around now.

Chapter Twenty

Marie was at school, having returned from Norman. She had prepared for her classes before she took her trip. Walking on air, Marie still enjoyed her teaching, but was getting anxious to get on with her move. It would be a big change for her, since she lived in the same apartment for thirteen years. The first things she thought of was Ted wouldn't be able to find her if he came back; but he had been gone for two years and it was time to give up on him. She considered what Dave told her about the economics of the move, but she still wanted to do it.

A couple of weeks after her visit to Dave, she prepared two of her favorite casseroles and called him up, "Hey, Dave, I've made some food and I wondered if I could come down and see you tomorrow."

"No."

"Are you busy? Would there be a better time?"

"No, you can't visit any time."

"But, David, you told me to come and see you whenever I wanted to. What happened?"

"Nothing happened. I just spoke out of turn."

"What do you mean?"

"I have a girlfriend here. I can't have you visit and I really don't want to talk to you again."

Marie choked back a tear. "Okay, I'll leave you alone then. Bye."

"Good bye."

Marie had her hopes up and she wished that David had told her that he had a girlfriend the weekend she was at his house. It would have been kinder. He treated her so well it had caught her off-guard. She guessed that would be the only time her boots would be warmed for her.

There was only a month to go at school. Most of her students were doing well, but Angela was unhappy. She wanted to go to school in San Antonio, but the school she applied to notify her there were no more dorm rooms. She was disappointed, because she was set on going to that particular school.

Marie liked Angela and her whole family. The family had her over for dinner and they were friendly to her. Marie really enjoyed herself with them. She wanted to help Angela and thought she could. Her brother, Tim, was a professor at the college Angela was interested in.

Marie called him up, and said, “Hey Tim, I have this student who really wants to go to your school but they are telling her that she can’t have a dorm room. She is only seventeen so she can’t live in an apartment, but is very intelligent and really wants to go to school there. Her parents also have a lot of pull. They own the Gallery.”

“For a student like her and on your recommendation,” he answered, “I’ll bet we can find a dorm room. I’ll talk to the Dean and have him call Angela’s parents.”

A few days later, Angela’s mother called Marie up. “Marie, I want to thank you and your brother for helping Angela get into the school we wanted her to go to. We are all just thrilled. Thank you so much.”

Marie would miss “her kids” but the truth of the matter was that she could not afford to teach at a job that paid so little, and besides, she was enamored with the idea of moving to Norman. Somehow, she knew that her life would be simpler and she would just get along much better in the smaller town she had loved when she was in college.

Marie felt hopeful about the future and was pleased when, at the last staff meeting, the Johnsons announced, "Guess what? Everyone is getting a $1,000 bonus in your last check!"

That really made all the hard work of the year seem worth it. Marie told them "I can't come back next year, I am moving out of town, but I enjoyed teaching here."

Graduation came, and Carolyn's father escorted her to the ceremony. Marie loved seeing the kids she worked with all year graduate and hearing their college plans. Not all of them, of course, were making plans for college, but those who were beamed.

A couple of days later, Marie received her last check in the mail. To her surprise, there was no sign of the bonus she expected. She called up Lloyd, the owner of the school, to see what happened. He said, "Marie, we thought we had already paid you enough."

Marie, confused and hurt, mumbled something like, "Oh, I see," and hung up. She cried, wondering why she was the only one who didn't get the bonus or so she assumed. Marie thought hadn't worked hard enough, or they didn't think she did a good enough job. Much later, Marie realized that since she wasn't returning to work the next year, they probably thought they could just save the money by not paying her.

Now it was really time to get out of town.

Marie asked her mother to help her find an apartment. They drove to Norman and began the search. There were only a few apartments in Marie's price range, most of them not very nice, even though it was the beginning of summer. They were pricey, since the town grew by 25,000 when school was in session. They finally found a decent duplex that allowed pets and that Marie could afford. It was small, with thin red carpeting and dull, off-white paint. The kitchen was standard apartment style, with old appliances in avocado green. However, the neighbor didn't look too neat. A pile of old, moldy bamboo shades was piled on the porch, looking like they had been there for months. Anyway, Marie rented it on the spot, though she had to call up the landlady and say, "I got the key to your apartment from the rental agent and looked at it. I would like to rent it."

The landlady said, "Leave a check for the deposit and the first month's rent and you can move in any time."

It seemed odd to not meet the landlady, but she had the apartment. She just returned home to start packing.

But before she started packing, she wrote a letter to her major professor at OU, who gave her so many chances to succeed fifteen years before. He let her into the Master's program when women weren't admitted, and he gave her a full scholarship to graduate school. Within a couple of days, he wrote her back, telling her to call him at home or at work, and giving her both numbers. So Marie felt like she had something set up, even if David was out as a lover.

Since she had been in that apartment so long, packing became a big sorting job. She threw out things like her high school yearbooks—what good were those? It took her a week, but she finally got everything all boxed up. She asked the couple who lived next door, Denise and Jim, "How would you like to make some money?"

She and the couple had lives next door to each other for two years. Denise was a short blond who was cute and Jim was a huge black man. Denise and Marie shared a love for cats and took care of each other's cats when one of them went out of town.

Denise had confided in her that she was an ex-prostitute and Jim used to be her pimp. She now worked at a Waffle House as a waitress and was much happier.

When Marie asked if they wanted to make extra money, Denise said, "How?"

Marie said, "I need someone to help me load the rental truck and drive it to Norman and unload it there. I'll pay you to help me."

Denise said, "That sounds like a good deal to me as long as it is on my day off."

"We'll arrange it that way." Marie was going to miss her nice apartment, but things were changing in her neighborhood. When she moved in, it was kind of shabby. Now it had become a desirable neighborhood and was being rehabbed. Gays were moving in and were fixing it up. The newer move-ins expected nicer apartments. Marie's rent had gone up $100 in the past six months after the building was painted inside and out.

Early in the morning on the day she was moving they started out: Marie in the car with the cats, and Denise and Jim following in the truck. When they got there, Marie stepped out of the car and looked around, puzzled. Something was wrong. Finally, it hit her. "Denise, look, my air conditioner has disappeared."

"Oh no, and it is already hot."

"Since it is Sunday, there's nothing to be done today. Let's unload and I'll unpack; I'll call the landlady tomorrow."

It was hot, so Denise and Jim were in a hurry to get back in the truck. "We can help you with the furniture but then we have to get back home." They unloaded in record time and returned to the City. Marie was left with a pile of unpacking to do.

Marie unpacked while the cats explored. Of course, they were not happy. Cats are never happy with change. Marie got everything unpacked just about the time it got dark.

The next day was spent getting the utilities turned on, water, gas, electricity, and phone. She had arranged them by phone previously and sent in the deposits, but it still took all day and wasn't fun. She called the landlady, but had to leave a message. "The air conditioner that was in the window when I rented the place is not there now. I guess it has been stolen. Please replace when you can. It is already hot, and I know it is going to get hotter."

That night she called Dr. Douglas, her major professor, at home. His wife answered, and when she asked for him, his wife asked, "Who are you?"

Marie said, "I am one of his old students, just moved back to town, and he told me to call him."

"Oh no, he didn't, he did not tell you to call him at his home. You are not to call him again here!"

Marie was embarrassed and somewhat ashamed. Not so much that she didn't call and leave a message on his office voicemail, but when he didn't return her call she didn't track him down in his office. He might have been a good source for a job, but Marie was too embarrassed to follow up.

She got up late the next day, and worked around the apartment before taking a walk to the campus, only a few blocks away. Marie looked around, happy to be in the small town again. She stopped to watch the hawks gliding in the sky over the river. The wind always blew in Oklahoma, and hawks all over the state took advantage of the currents.

Marie went to her favorite place on campus, the library. It was a huge, gothic-style building with lots of woodwork and it housed over a million books. It was also air-conditioned, and when Marie went to school there, it was the only building with that amenity.

She really didn't think she could get a library card since she wasn't a student or an employee of the college, but she asked anyway. "What do you have to do to get a library card?"

The clerk answered, "You have to be a student, an employee, or you have to have a need to have a card."

“Oh, well then, I qualify. Is my drivers’ license what you need for ID?”

“What kind of need do you have?”

“I will simply go crazy if I live this close to so many books and I am not allowed to use them.”

“Sounds right to me.”

The clerk checked her ID and issued Marie a temporary library card. Marie wandered around in the stacks and found several books to read. Then she hurried home .She went to bed early with a book, after calling the landlady again. “I see that you didn’t install my air conditioner today. I know it takes time to get one and have it installed, but it is really warm in here.”

Actually, it was mid-June and she could easily handle the nights by simply opening the windows, but she didn’t want the landlady to forget about her. The next morning Marie called her again, and got her this time.

She said, “My air conditioner was stolen before I moved in. It’s really hot in here.”

The landlady, not sounding concerned at all, said, “Okay, I’ll take care of it. You’ll have a new air conditioner tomorrow.”

Chapter Twenty-One

To Marie's great surprise, the next morning a truck drove up and a man got out, came to the door, and said, "I'm here to install your new air conditioner."

"Well, it is about time. I have called the landlady a dozen times."

Within a few minutes, it felt a lot better in the apartment. The cats even perked up. Marie spent the day reading, but the whole time she could feel time clicking by. She wasn't looking for work and her savings were slipping away. She resolved to start looking for work the next day.

When she walked to the campus to get the paper, she stopped to watch the hawks circling over the river. It was always one of her favorite sights. They were hunting, and looked like they didn't have a care in the world as they glided on the wind.

She got the local newspaper, but was not surprised there were no appropriate jobs advertised in it. In a town like Norman, employers didn't need to advertise for professionals—they had their pick. Marie tried the personnel office at the University. Few jobs were listed; she remembered what Dave said about a hiring freeze. There was one opening for a financial aid officer.

Marie didn't like the sound of that—it seemed a lot like Food Stamps. However, she was not in a position to be choosy, so she took an application with her and filled it out at home. Marie returned it to the office the next day, confident this was a job she could do and would get.

She got a call for an interview to be set up for the next week.

Meanwhile, she was making friends with some of the people in the neighborhood. One woman, Evelyn, came to see her every day. She was in her thirties, brown-haired and attractive, unemployed, and, like Marie, just moved back to Norman. They would talk about the news of the day and their lives. They were sitting in the living room by the air conditioner when Marie asked her, "Evelyn, how do you make a living?"

"I enter contests and I pay my bills when I win one."

Marie thought that sounded odd, but couldn't get her to explain further.

She also met students at the library who were hanging around Norman between semesters or going to summer school. They treated her like a friend, not an old lady. Marie felt like she should be going to school, too, but didn't know how to afford it. If she got on the staff at OU, then she would get a big discount on her tuition and could take a few classes.

Marie knew how to get a job; she'd done it plenty of times. Show up, dressed to the nines and on time for the scheduled interview. They started off by asking her, "So, you were a student here back in the Sixties?"

"Yes, and I loved it here. I wanted to move back here and work for the University. I have nothing but good memories of the school and the town."

"You have never worked for a Financial Aid Office, but it looks like you have had several similar jobs."

"Yes, Marie said, "I have worked for Food Stamps and the Police Department certifying people for benefits. I think that would be the same sort of job as a Financial Aid Officer, but of course I would be working here, where I want to work."

She thought the interview was going well, but she couldn't help but notice that the interviewers, a Dean and the head of Financial Aid, kept giving each other looks over her head. It seemed like they didn't believe her or they didn't quite understand what she was saying. Marie didn't know what was going on, but it didn't look good. Marie left the interview with less confidence than when she came in. She wished she could have asked them what was wrong.

Marie checked the jobs board on-campus daily and kept looking at the ads in the paper, both the local Norman paper and the campus paper, but nothing turned up. After a couple of weeks, she got a letter from the Financial Aid Office, saying, "We are happy that you applied for the position of Financial Aid Officer, but unfortunately we have chosen another applicant who we believe is better suited for the position."

Marie got a little panicky then. That was the only job in a month that she was eligible to apply for. The next day, racking her brain, she thought about going to school full time and getting a grant to do so. She went to the Admissions Office and asked the woman in charge, "How would I get a grant or loan to go to school in the fall?"

"We give you aid based on the income you had last year."

"But I don't have access to my last year's income. I spent it last year. Now I don't have any income."

"We don't figure your income that way."

"In the Sixties, I never ran into that because I was always broke."

"I'm just telling you what the rules are."

"But that makes me ineligible for the help I need."

"I'm sorry," said the administrator.

Marie went home, with an option she thought was open to her closed off.

She was rapidly running out of options. There were other jobs, minimum-wage jobs, open to the students. She found one stacking books in the library. That was her job when she was a student at the University, so she had experience. Managing to get an interview for that one, she walked to the library the day of the interview. The lady in the little book-covered office was younger than she was and seemed skeptical from the start.

Marie said, "I came back to the University in order to take some classes and I thought I could get a job stacking books just as I did when I was a student. I have years of experience and really know what I am doing."

"Even though you have an MA, you wouldn't mind stacking books for a living again?"

"Oh, no, that would be fine with me as long as I got to take classes."

The lady didn't buy it

At home, Marie stopped turning on the air conditioner to save money. She sat around in the heat, trying to figure out what to do. Evelyn kept encouraging her to turn on the air conditioner, and it made Marie think that was why she had been visiting her every day.

She couldn't even concentrate enough to watch TV. Obviously, David had been straight with her about the economy. She wanted to live in Norman, still considering it the best place to be, but she had to find a way to make a living.

About six weeks after she moved there, worried and anxious as she searched for openings every morning but didn't find anything, she was out doing errands in her beat-up old copper-colored Mustang, when suddenly she found herself driving aggressively, as if she were full of rage. She was pulling at the wheel and rolling over the railroad tracks at full speed. Anyone observing her would think she was in the throes of road rage.

At the same time, she calmly thought, Weird—I'm driving like an idiot and I don't feel the slightest bit upset. There is something definitely wrong here, and I don't know what it is. She was detached from how she was acting. She felt nothing like her actions portrayed.

When she got home, without thinking about it, or considering how she felt about counseling, she pulled out the Norman phone book and looked up "Mental Health Center."

She told the woman who answered what she had told herself minutes before, "There is something wrong with me and I don't know what it is."

"Could you be more specific?"

"No, I can't. I was just driving like a maniac and I didn't have any reason to be doing that. I can't explain it."

"Is this an emergency? Do you feel like doing harm to yourself?"

"No, I don't feel like that."

"We can give you an appointment in ten days, August 12, at 11 a.m.

"That will be fine."

After the call and getting the appointment, Marie felt some relief, but she didn't monitor her feelings or try to figure out what was going on with her. One thing that stood out was that she had brought a good supply of marijuana with her so she would be able to sleep, but it stopped working. No matter how much she smoked, she couldn't sleep at night. She decided she must have gotten a bad batch. She went to some of her young friends and asked, "Do you want this lid? I really don't anymore."

One of them said, "Sure!"

A couple of days later, when they saw Marie again, he said, "Hey thanks. That's some really good stuff."

That puzzled Marie, but she didn't think much more about it. In fact, she wasn't thinking or feeling much at all. She was just sort of vegetating, not eating much as she didn't have an appetite. She was just waiting for her appointment. For some reason, after all that time of not believing that counseling could help, she was looking forward to this appointment as something important to her life.

She hadn't told her parents about it because she didn't think they would approve. They believed that if you had a mental problem or a nervous one, the best way to handle it was to suck up and manage it, not start blabbing it to strangers. In fact, they did not really believe in mental problems, they were "just in your head." Therefore, she did not think that she could ask them for advice or help. She just waited for the appointment, almost incuriously. It was un-Marie-like.

Chapter Twenty-Two

The day of the appointment Marie wasn't really nervous, just a little anxious, since she didn't know what to expect. She just hoped they could help her. The clinic was all the way across town and she left about a half-hour early to make her appointment on time. It was kind of embarrassing when her arrival time was nine minutes.

The clinic was new, and pleasant-looking, small, faced with white trim. Marie went into a small waiting room with a secretary working at a typewriter. She approached her and said, "I have an eleven o'clock appointment. I'm sorry to be so early but I just moved here from the City and I'm not used to getting around in such a small town."

The young secretary, brushed a ringlet of red hair aside, laughed, and said, "Don't worry, it happens all the time. Just have a seat and Dr. Craig will be with you in a minute."

Marie sat for about twenty minutes, but finally Dr. Craig, a young man in his early thirties, came out of his office. He was tall, with brown hair and eyes.

"Marie? Please come into my office."

Marie went in and sat down. Dr. Craig said, "I don't know much about why you are here. Could you tell me a little bit about yourself?"

There was so much to tell. Marie said, speaking rapidly, "Well, first off I went with this guy for ten years—we never had that good a relationship—but then he dumped me and left without even telling me goodbye. I had a job with the Police Department but I quit that one, and then I got on with Food

Stamps where I worked seven years, but I lost that one. Then I got a job as a teacher in a private school but that one wasn't enough to pay the bills and everything just got harder and harder so I decided to move to Norman. I went to school here fifteen years ago and I know what a nice town this is to live in. I was hoping to find a job and maybe go to school part time, but I haven't been able to find a thing and now my money is running out. Then two weeks ago, I was driving too fast and erratically, I don't know why. The fact of the matter is that I can't do anything right."

"Now you are being ridiculous. You have both shoes on, and they match. You made it to the appointment on time and by yourself. You are catastrophizing. It's not as bad as you think it is," he said.

"Why was I driving the car as if I were a maniac the other day? It was scary."

"I have a theory about that. I think you made up your mind that if you didn't find a job you would have to kill yourself. Now you don't have a job and you're running out of money, so your back is to the wall and you think your only solution is to commit suicide. You are panicking."

"Oh, is that what's happening? It makes sense. I don't see any way out."

"There are plenty of options. You just need to be able to see them. I think you are an endogenous depressive, which means that depression comes from the inside, not from any outside occurrence. I am going to prescribe an antidepressant for you, hoping that it helps to change your outlook"

"Doctor," said Marie, "I have another problem. I don't sleep. For the past ten years, I have smoked marijuana to help me sleep, but the last few weeks it hasn't worked anymore. I am utterly exhausted."

"The first thing for you to do is to stop smoking marijuana. It interferes with the medication I am going to give you. It is a depressive, so it can't help you. You'll find that the medicine I give you will make you sleep—you will probably sleep all day tomorrow."

"That sounds good. I'll try the antidepressant if you think it will help."

"Yes, I do, and I want you to talk to a Social Worker twice a week. My secretary makes the appointments. I'll call and ask the woman who handles the medications to wait a few minutes so you don't have to come back after lunch."

"Thank you, Dr. Craig, I appreciate that.

"Okay, make your appointments and pick up your meds. I'll see you next week. Bye."

After she made appointments with the Social Worker and another one with Dr. Craig, she got directions to the medication clinic. "Wait a minute," said the secretary. "Do you know what Dr. Craig did the first time he went to a movie here after moving from Dallas?"

Marie shook her head.

"He and his wife showed up at the movie theatre so early they hadn't opened the box office yet!" They laughed together and Marie headed for the next-door pharmacy clinic, where the pharmacist already had her meds ready. She asked, "Do you have a job?"

Marie said "No."

Then she asked, "What are you living on?"

Marie explained, "I have some savings from my last job."

"Then these won't cost you anything. Let me know if you have any difficulty with them, and be careful. Only take the prescribed amount. Too many can kill you. "

Marie thanked her and left, a little wary of the pills she held in her hand.

Marie went straight home and immediately took one of her pills. They were the latest in antidepressants and Dr. Craig had told her they would take about ten days to work. She put the pill bottle in the bathroom and every time she walked into the room it was to feel a little frisson of fear—she thought it was because she knew it was possible to commit suicide with the pills and she was a little afraid she might do it.

After a while, she got sleepy and went to bed. That night she slept all night and the next day, she woke up only a few times. She got up long enough to eat a sandwich and to take another pill.

Marie was wakened by the phone in the evening. It was her mother calling. Marie could hardly put a coherent sentence together. Her mother had arranged a picnic in a park in Norman for the next day with her sisters Shirley and Ann, who was in town, and her aunt Clarice. She wanted to alert Marie as to when and where it was.

Marie, haltingly and slowly, told her mother she couldn't attend. "Mother, I went to the doctor and he gave me some pills. I can hardly stay awake and I certainly can't drive."

"What is wrong with you?"

Not willing to open up to her mother completely, Marie replied, "Well, he thinks I might be a little depressed so he gave me some antidepressants to see how I react. Mostly I have been groggy, but I've only taken them for two days."

"You sure sound groggy. Are you certain you are all right?"

"Yes, he said that I would react this way at first," Marie said.

"Ann and Shirley are coming to the picnic and I know Aunt Clarice wants to see you, so I will come by and pick you up about eleven."

"Mother, I told you I am all groggy."

"You'll be fine. You need someone to bring you food, anyway."

Marie felt somewhat better in the morning, though her speech was still slow and slurred, and she had some trouble walking. She was able to get dressed, but when her mother and sister Ann arrived, they had to help her into the car.

They had the picnic in a park, eating on a stone WPA picnic table under a huge elm. It was pleasant in the shade, with the birds singing, but Marie felt like she was wrapped in gelatin. She wanted to talk to everyone, but it seemed so difficult. She was especially happy to see her Aunt Clarice, who she hadn't seen in a few years. When she and Shirley were young, they used to spend parts of the summer at Uncle Joe's and Aunt Clarice's farm, swimming in the ponds, eating the best fried chicken, and helping with the chores they were able to handle. Aunt Clarice was good to them and they always loved her for it.

Now she really couldn't talk to her, she was just able to say, "Aunt Clarice, I am happy to see you. How are Uncle Joe and the farm? I hope you are feeling well."

Aunt Clarice said, "Well, I wanted to have this picnic because I heard you were in Norman and it is easier for me to drive here than to the City from the farm. But my goodness, girl, what is wrong with you?"

Marie said, "I took some pills, and they made me groggy."

Her aunt was too polite to ask for details. Marie was able to eat, and her sister Shirley had made her favorite dish. She hadn't eaten much in the past two days, so the food seemed particularly good.

She had to be helped to and from the car and was embarrassed by her condition. It was good seeing everyone but she wished she were in shape to interact with her relatives.

When they left, she said, "Goodbye, everyone. I hope the next time I see you I am more conscious."

Her mother and Ann drove her home and her mother helped her into the house. She asked again, "Are you sure you are okay? Those pills seem awfully strong."

"Mother, he said they would take a while for me to get used to them. I promise I'll call him if I don't get better by tomorrow."

"You do that and I'll call you tomorrow to see how you are doing."

Marie noticed, just barely, as she walked in the front door that the pile of stuff on the on the neighbor's porch had disappeared and the porch was cleaned up. That was some good news.

Chapter Twenty-Three

The next morning Marie woke up feeling much better and much sharper. Her mother called and asked, "How are you doing?"

Marie was able to answer her in an almost clear voice, "I feel much more human today. I think I am getting used to these pills. Thanks for taking me to the picnic yesterday. The food was good and I enjoyed seeing everyone."

After Marie hung up, she remembered it was her day to meet with the Social Worker and got dressed for the appointment. At the office, she didn't have to wait long for the counselor. Alice was a pleasant, attractive young woman.

"My husband and I are from New York City," Alice said. "He is studying meteorology in grad school so of course we had to come to OU. The first nights we were here we kept hearing this funny noise. Neither of us knew what it was and it kind of scared me. It turned out to be the cattle lowing. I'd never heard anything like that."

Marie laughed at the story and felt at ease.

"Now I know how you are now; what about your early life?"

"My father was dominant and unpredictable. We never knew what to expect from him or who he was going to be. My mother was always loving and caring. She really made it possible for us to grow up halfway sane. I don't know what it is, but there is something definitely wrong with my family. One time, when I was twelve, my father kicked me out of the house. I just kept a low profile until my mother came home."

Alice said, "The problem could be inherited, and you could have good reason to be depressed. Do you feel any better?"

Marie told her, "I feel better now that I am sleeping, but I don't feel my depression lifting."

Alice reassured her, "It will probably be another week before you feel the effects of the antidepressants."

Their session over, Marie went home feeling better about herself. For the first time, she thought she might actually be getting some help. When she got home, she parked her car in front. She was walking up the sidewalk to her apartment when she suddenly felt little bugs jumping on her feet and legs. "What the hell?" She asked herself.

When she got inside, she investigated the situation and discovered that fleas had taken over the front yard and had jumped from the yard to her feet and legs. Her ankles were covered with them. Marie was horrified and shuddered. One year her family had come home from vacation and discovered that fleas had invaded the house. Marie remembered how awful it was until they could get an exterminator in. Her ankles started to itch.

Marie grabbed the phone and called the landlady. She told her about the fleas. The landlady asked her what made her think there were fleas on the lawn. Marie was close to tears already and started to get hysterical.

"I know because they were jumping on my legs as I walked up the sidewalk. This has to be taken care of now—or they will be in the house and on my cats and I just can't take that. I think it happened when my neighbor cleaned her porch."

The landlady said, "How do you know that it wasn't caused by your cats?"

"I just had them to the vet for their shots and he will certify that they didn't have fleas then.

"Well, if you are sure it is a problem, call a pest control company and have them come out and treat the lawn for fleas and send the bill to me. But I am going to check with them and make sure there were fleas there."

Marie said, "I promise there are fleas all over the front yard."

Marie was relieved that she finally got some help from the landlady, but by the time she got the go-ahead to call an exterminator she was crying, and upset. She got ahold of one and the girl who answered the phone, without putting her on "hold" simply yelled out, "Hey, I got a crazy lady on one."

Marie slammed down the phone, crying harder. She decided she had better compose herself before going any further. She gave herself a couple of minutes, then called another company and made an appointment for the next morning. The exterminator men came the next day and treated the lawn and got rid of the fleas. Marie was glad that had been taken care of so easily, but she was still bitten badly.

That afternoon, she was surprised to see her mother and father drive up. They hadn't called first, they just showed up. Her father thought her landlady did not cut the grass often enough. Once before he had brought his mower and cut her grass, even though it didn't bother Marie and she didn't care how long the grass was. She had a lot more on her mind than the condition of the lawn. Because he was unhappy with the junk on her neighbor's porch, he threatened not to mow her half of the lawn. Marie said, "Please, don't get me in a fight with my neighbor."

Thankfully, he went ahead and mowed the whole lawn.

This time her father didn't even come in the house or greet her. He just pulled the mower out of the trunk of the car and prepared to cut the grass. Marie saw this and said to Susie, who had come into the house to talk with her, "Mother, will you go out and ask him not to cut the grass too short because it was just treated for fleas and I don't want to lose all the chemicals."

She sent her mother because she knew that no matter what she tried to say to her father, it would not go over well.

"Okay," her mother said and went outside and talked with him. In a few minutes she returned and told Marie, "I made a mistake."

"What do you mean, you made a mistake?"

"I must have told him wrong because he got mad and now he says we have to go home."

"Mother, you didn't make a mistake. It's his problem. If he can't handle a simple request then let him be mad. And don't let him take it out on you."

Marie's mother hurried outside and got in the car. Her father peeled out, never having said a word to Marie. She was so angry. It was just another case of his unpredictability, which all of the kids had lived with their whole lives.

The next day, Marie had a brainstorm. She went to the OU library and found the section on depression. There were dozens of books for her to peruse. She wanted to learn all she could about this disease she had been diagnosed with. She gathered some of the more interesting-looking ones, then checked the job bulletin boards. Nothing available in the way of jobs, so she headed home and spent the next couple of days immersed in her reading.

The reading was interesting and she learned a lot, but it all boiled down to taking your medicine and something called cognitive behavior therapy, what Dr. Craig and Alice were practicing on her—trying to change her negative thinking to a more positive slant.

She read all she could and much of the behavior of her family was explained to her. After about a week some of her new friends stopped by to ask her if she wanted to go to a movie with them.

"Sure," she said, and put on some makeup to get ready. They walked to the theatre, and when they got there, she realized that this was the first time in months she felt like doing something for fun. And felt like putting on makeup. My goodness, she did feel better! She was suddenly conscious that she felt much more confident and joyful than she had in years. It was a major change.

Two days later, at an appointment with Dr. Craig, Alice was in the waiting room when she got there. “How are you feeling?”

Marie threw her arms around Alice and said, “I feel wonderful!”

Dr. Craig walked in and Marie saw him exchange a glance with Alice.

He asked Marie to come into his office. When they were settled he said, “I see the antidepressants are starting to work.”

“Oh, yes, I feel so much better. The change is amazing.”

“Have you made any plans?”

“Yes, Doctor, in the past few days I have been thinking that I am wasting my time and money staying here in Norman. I’m getting nowhere. I think I should return to the City, where I can always find work.”

“I think that is a good idea. I will give you plenty of meds and a letter to give to your new doctor with my observations. When will you move?”

“Just as soon as I can make arrangements. Maybe in a week or two. I’ll let you know.”

“Just call and tell me the date and I’ll have the letter and the medication ready for you. I think you are doing the right thing,” Dr. Craig said.

They talked a little longer about how Marie felt and the change that had come over her, then Marie talked with Alice for a while.

“Alice, I’ve decided to move back to the City. I can’t find a job here and I know I can get something there. I will miss living in Norman but I am just running through my money here."

"Marie, you are really feeling a lot better and I see change. I think you have made the right decision."

Alice gave her some ideas about trying to stay busy when she was depressed—something like taking a walk or cleaning out a closet. She said that activity would help to keep her from brooding. Before she left for home, Alice said, "I hope I see you again before you leave."

That evening a cold front blew in from the north. Summer was ending and Marie needed heat. The apartment furnace was broken, and had been since she moved in. The landlady promised to fix it before it got cold, but now it was cold and she had no heat. Marie called her several times, asking, "when are you going to fix the furnace?" All she got were promises.

Finally, Marie found the Tenant's Union in the phone book, and called them. It turned out they were set up to protect students from predatory landlords. She told the guy on the phone, "Hey, I'm cold and I don't have any heat."

He said, "Who is your landlord?"

Marie said, "Ms. Martin."

"Oh, she knows better than that. I'll give her a call and I guarantee you will have heat tomorrow."

"I didn't know it was so easy, or I would have done this a long time ago."

The man showed up the next day to repair her furnace.

Chapter Twenty-Four

Marie drove into town to talk with her parents.

"Mother, she said, "what do you think I should do? I know I need to move but it is so expensive. What do you think is the best way for me to go?"

Her father, who was in the living room reading the paper, spoke up, "You can rent a truck and Paul and I will move you."

"Oh no, that is way too much for you. I can't let you do that. I just thought you might know some people who did moves."

"Don't be ridiculous—of course we'll move you. You and your mother can find a new apartment and then we'll pack you up and get you moved."

Marie knew there was no turning them down now. Her father had his mind made up. "Wow, that's great. I'll start looking for a place tomorrow"

The next day Marie looked for an apartment, but not in the same neighborhood. When she first moved into her old neighborhood, thirteen years ago, it was kind of old and picturesque. Over the years, it had gained in personality, and become a revitalized area. The majority of its residents were now gay. Shortly before she moved, her rent had gone up a hundred dollars a month and it was obvious she couldn't stay because it was becoming too expensive.

This time she looked in the far north part of the City, where twenty years ago, new singles apartment complexes had sprung up. Now they were somewhat shabby. She quickly found a place, one that would take her cats and rent was much lower than the old neighborhood.

Before she did anything else, Marie called Dr. Craig.

"Doctor, I'll be moving soon. What do I need to do?"

"Good, I'm glad you are making plans to get back to your life. Just stop by anytime during working hours and my secretary has a letter for you to take to your new doctor. Also, I left orders with the pharmacy to have two months of antidepressants ready for you to pick up, so you'll have time to get started with the Mental Health Center up there."

"Thank you Dr. Craig. You have made my life so much easier and better."

"I enjoyed working with you, but you have a big challenge ahead. Just stay on your medication and keep trying."

"I will. I want to thank you and Alice for all your help."

Back at her duplex, Marie started packing, muttering to herself, "What kind of idiot moves every couple of months? There isn't anything worse than moving, and I am making it into a hobby."

About that time, her mother called. "How is it going?"

"I have an apartment rented and started packing. I've wound things up with the doctor so will be ready to go in a few days. It just depends on when you can help me."

"I'll talk to Daddy and see what he wants to do. I'm glad you are moving back to town."

Marie decided the most important thing on her list was to get her letter and pills from the clinic, so she hurried there and picked them up. She was a little frightened about starting a new life, but not nearly so scared as she was when realizing the dead end facing her just a few weeks ago...

Marie spent all her time packing, and was ready to go in four days. Meanwhile, her father said he could move her as soon as she got packed. On Tuesday, Marie rented a U-Haul truck and she, her father, and Uncle Paul loaded the truck and made their way to her new apartment. Then it was just a case of unloading and unpacking. Mother had driven their car to the apartment so she stayed to help her unpack, and Peter and Paul went home to have a drink and rest. "Thank you so much for moving me. That made everything so much easier. Now I just have to start looking for a job. I do appreciate it."

Marie was tense with her father there; she never knew what would set him off. Her mother and she could relax and unpack with just the two of them there. It went fast and Marie drove her mother home after a couple of hours so her father wouldn't get upset at her absence. "Thank you, Mother, for all your help and for keeping things calm. This was one of the easiest moves of my life and I hope I don't move again for a long time."

"I was happy to help you. I wanted you back in town"

After her parents left, Marie sat down to rest. She felt guilty because she allowed her parents to work so hard. However, they seemed not to mind, and it saved her lots of money when she didn't really have much. She watched the cats tentatively and unhappily explore their new home.

She finished setting up the apartment the next day, and started looking for a job the day after. An advertisement in the paper sounded promising, so she called up and made an appointment for an interview.

When she got to the address, it was in a strip mall and she was applying at a trade school—The Mid-Cities Training Academy, The job was as "registrar" of the school but it was really as a secretary. They just needed her graduate degree to look good for the accreditors.

The salary was enough to keep her alive and the work was certainly not onerous. Marie took the job knowing she could keep looking while she worked. As Marie got to know the workings of the school, she was not impressed with the education they offered. They trained medical assistants, paralegal assistants, and several other fields. The teachers did not seem professional when she interacted with them, the school's "representatives" were only interested in how many sales they could make, and the boss seemed a bit "off." He was brash and fired people periodically for reasons Marie couldn't fathom. He seemed to enjoy it. She kept to herself and just tried to do the work well.

Marie worked there for several months when the forecast for the next day was" icy precipitation." She told Frank, the boss, that if the roads were bad the next morning she wouldn't be in because it was scary to drive when it was slippery. He was from Kansas City, and he said that anyone who didn't come in the next day was automatically fired. Marie had spent two years in college close to Kansas City, and she knew they did not know much about ice there—it generally snowed.

When Marie woke up the next morning, an inch of ice covered the streets. Marie fired up the car and got out on the street, but she couldn't control the car. Luckily, few people were trying to drive. After half a mile of hitting curbs and running off the road, Marie turned the car around and went home. She tried for the next two days to call into work, but couldn't reach anyone. On the third day, the streets were better, so she went in, halfway expecting to be fired. Frank said nothing, except that he hadn't been in either for the past two days. The subject was never brought up again.

Meanwhile, Marie had worked quickly to find a new doctor. It was several weeks before she could get an appointment, but Dr. Craig had given her extra meds in case that happened. The Mental Health Center was the same one she went to for counseling several years before. It was located near downtown, in kind of a seedy area. Two bus lines converged here, which was one reason for the clinic's location.

When she arrived, about thirty people waited to be seen. The building was low and squat, made of dark red brick. Inside, it was depressingly dark, but she did note there was now a pharmacy window in the lobby. That seemed like an improvement.

Marie made the appointment for the evening so she wouldn't miss any work. The receptionist, who was seated behind bulletproof glass, surprised her by going out of her way to be rude. Marie felt herself getting tense, wondering what her new doctor was like, and what the letter she held in her hand said.

Chapter Twenty-Five

Dr. Kruger was elderly, grizzled with grey hair and a beard, and was overweight. After Marie told him she was diagnosed with endogenous depression in Norman and the type of antidepressant she was taking, he opened the letter Dr. Craig gave her.

"This is interesting," Kruger said. "Dr. Craig thinks, because of your reaction to the antidepressant, you should be diagnosed with bipolar disorder and treated accordingly."

"No, he didn't." Marie said, shocked. "That is not what he told me." She did all that research on depression, but knew next to nothing about bipolar disorder.

"Here, see for yourself." The doctor handed her the letter,

"Marie became manic after the administration of a course of antidepressants, and it is my opinion that she suffers from bipolar disorder and should be treated as such."

"I don't believe it." she said, convinced the first diagnosis was the correct one,

Dr. Kruger said, "This is a common finding, and it doesn't surprise me. Let's at least proceed as if Dr. Craig is correct. You trust him, don't you?

"Yes, I do trust his judgment. I'll at least try what you recommend."

"Lithium is the treatment of choice for bipolar disorder, so I'll start you on that immediately."

"What about the antidepressants?"

"Lithium takes care of that, but I'll continue you on them until the lithium takes hold. You'll be amazed at how fast it works. Don't be afraid; bipolar disorder is easy to control. All you have to do is to take your medication."

"I'm glad to hear that. I'm feeling so much better since I started on the other meds."

"You can get your lithium at the pharmacy downstairs. Make an appointment with the appointment desk in two weeks and we'll see how you are doing."

"Thank you, Doctor."

Marie turned in her prescription and made her appointment with the receptionist, went to the pharmacy pick up her pills, then went back to the receptionist to pay, always waiting in long lines. All the bureaucracy took about an hour, but she finally was on the way home. She was still confused about her diagnosis; the antidepressants seemed to be working so well. She could not recall ever feeling as good as when she starting taking them.

Marie started the lithium the next morning and waited to see what would happen. There were no immediate side effects, in fact, no effects from the drug all week Maybe it would just take it a while to kick in.

On Saturday, she went to the downtown public library and found they had only one book on bipolar disorder. Thankfully, it was checked in. She started reading it as soon as she got home and finished that evening. It didn't help all that much. It emphasized such behavior as overspending, which was something that Marie had never done. It described people spending money they didn't have for things they didn't need and going into thousands of dollars of debt.

Sure, Marie might buy four lipsticks instead of one, but she had never gone into debt for anything except a car. A bipolar person didn't seem to do things that she did, according to this book. She was even more confused when finishing reading it than when starting it. It did describe people who did things on impulse and used bad judgment. Marie could see that she did that sometimes, but she couldn't identify any extreme behavior.

When she returned to the Clinic after two weeks, the doctor asked her, "How do you feel?"

"Exactly as I did before. No change.'

"Are you sure?"

"Yes, I'm sure. The lithium had no effect on me at all. I'm still dubious about my diagnosis."

Doctor Kruger said, "Haven't you had times when you were happier than other times and when you did things that didn't seem quite right? Bipolar disorder is known for lapses of judgment, hypersexuality, and impulsivity. After interacting with you, I'm fairly certain you are bipolar. However, you should have reacted to the medicine. I'll up the dosage and see you again in two weeks."

Marie went through the rigmarole to get her drugs and was again startled by the rude clerks. She wished she didn't have to come here but she knew something was wrong with her and wanted to get it under control. At this time, with no health insurance since her mental disorder was a pre-existing condition, she couldn't afford a private doctor or to buy drugs retail.

Marie tried to remember times when she might have been hypersexual or impulsive, or could have used bad judgment. She remembered the time hitchhikers, complete strangers, stayed in the house and the times she cheated on Ted, but none of it seemed extreme to her. That was just normal behavior to her, well, except maybe for the hitchhikers. That was a little extreme. And the time she threw the guy out of the apartment, because Ted called her while he was there. Maybe.

While she was trying to get her moods under control and not having any success, she still had to support herself. She was still working at the school as the "registrar." At work a fairly new employee, Bruce, was popular because of his good nature. He worked as a representative and was doing a good job. He called in sick for a couple of days and then came in with his leg in a cast and on crutches. When asked what happened, he said, “I fell and broke my ankle.”

Marie said, “How did that happen?”

“I’m not quite sure. One minute I was standing there, and the next I was on the ground.”

Everyone was properly sympathetic, but two weeks later, he didn’t come into work and he didn’t call. Finally, in the afternoon, he came in and seemed agitated. He needed to talk with Frank.

Marie heard him say, “Frank, I fell again, and for no reason. I didn’t trip, I wasn’t dizzy, I just fell. So I went to the doctor and he says I have a brain tumor. I have to fly to Virginia tomorrow morning for emergency surgery. Can the company help me with anything? I’m having trouble with the insurance.”

Frank said, “I am sorry to hear that. You start packing up your stuff and I’ll call human resources at the home office and see what I can find out.”

After a while, Frank called Bruce up to his office.

Bruce came out after a few minutes. He announced to no one in particular, “The company can’t help me because I am new and the tumor is a pre-existing condition. They are letting me go. But I am going to be fine, just fine. Frank tells me Jesus will take care of me.”

Bruce used his crutches to get out of the office as fast as he could. Marie’s felt a wave of nausea wash over her. She averted her eyes and tried not to show how upset she was. Everyone went back to work and Bruce was never mentioned again.

Marie wanted to quit after that, but she couldn’t. It wasn’t the principle of the thing, but the fact was that she needed the money too badly to leave. However, that quandary was solved for her soon; Frank came to work in an especially good mood one morning about a week later and fired Marie, giving her two weeks' notice. He gave no reason, and she didn't ask. She figured it was just like the others he fired. He just felt like it. So it was time to find another job; it didn't upset her as much this time.

Marie went to Kelly Girls and took their tests, doing well enough that she picked up short assignments right away. She didn't like finding a new office and working for new people and learning new rules and jobs every few weeks, but it was a living. Meanwhile, she looked for a real job.

After a while, Marie got on as a temporary worker with the City, the assignment she got was at, of all places, the sewage plant. The atmosphere was funny; everyone was standoffish. No one was nice to her.

When she met her new boss, all he said was. "You remind me of that girl in the movie 'Sweet November'."

Marie was startled. The movie was about a woman who slept with a different man every month. She didn't know why he would say something like that to her. She replied, "I don't look like her," she said, "and I certainly don't act like her."

Then Marie went back to work. (She did wonder if her reputation had preceded her, but didn't know how it could have.) A week or so later, she was late to work with some car trouble. The boss said, "I would have called you, but I thought you might be in bed with some man."

"You are my boss, so you had every right to call, no matter who I was in bed with," Marie said. Shrugging, went back to work.

Later that afternoon, while she was having lunch, the engineer who was second-in-command, George, sat down with her and told her why everyone was so unfriendly. "Everyone we get in here is so turned off by the boss' sexual harassment that we lose them right away. You seem to have confused him. He hasn't laid a hand on you, yet."

"Trust me, he won't," Marie replied.

Marie was able to work at that job for several months by simply ignoring what the boss said. He never worked up the courage to touch her. She had a short affair with George, who was married. Everyone at the plant and city personnel was happy with her, and she was able to stay on, even though the situation was not the best, and it was always tense.

Chapter Twenty-Six

ON Marie's next visit to the clinic, Dr. Kruger asked, "can you tell if the Lithium is helping?'

"No, I can't tell that it is making any difference at all. It has no effect except to make me gain weight."

"That is a side effect you will just have to get used to. But by this time and with this dosage you should be feeling the effects of the drug."

"I'm not. I don't feel any different at all," replied Marie.

"It is helping you. You just don't recognize it. I may not be a psychiatrist but I know how to treat bipolar disorder."

"You aren't a psychiatrist?"

"No, I was an orthopedic surgeon but I got arthritis in my hands, so I had to retire and take this job where I can treat patients without using my hands. But I have been doing this for years. Don't worry."

"If the lithium were helping, I would be able to tell. It is not doing anything, I tell you."

"Just keep taking it and soon you will see how much it helps you."

Marie was feeling nothing but frustration. All that hassle every time she needed to get more drugs, and yet they didn't seem to do anything but make her gain weight. The weight gain was already twenty pounds. Was she ever going to stop gaining weight? And why wasn't her doctor a psychiatrist? That didn't seem reasonable; it was a mental illness, she needed a doctor qualified to treat her.

With no regular work and living without friends in a new apartment complex, Marie was lonely. Also, taking antidepressants made her feel more like socializing. She tried joining a Bipolar Support Group, but everyone seemed so pitiful and felt sorry for themselves.

No matter what, Marie told herself, she wasn't going to be like that. She tried to bring a little humor, a little lightness into the group, but everyone seemed down all the time. There was always some reason why they would never be better. Finally, Marie connected with Pam; they talked together in a couple of meetings, and went for a coke afterwards. Then she picked up the newspaper one morning the next week and there was this story:

"Local Woman in Shoot-Out with Police"

Pam had locked herself in her home and called the police threatening to kill herself. When they arrived, she shot at them with a pistol—it sounded like an attempted case of suicide by cop. Luckily, everyone came out of it okay, but Marie never went back to a Support Group Meeting.

Then Marie ran across a mention of Mensa in a newspaper or magazine. That reminded her of high school, when IQ tests were administered and the principal of her school called in her parents. He told them, "Marie scored in the top two percent of the people in the country on her IQ test. I wanted you to know that because I think you should think about sending her to college." Her parents agreed, but had already told Marie her only hope for college was a scholarship.

The only criterion for joining Mensa was an IQ score in the top two percent of the population. That's something I can do to meet people, she thought. She dialed information for the number for the National Mensa Office in New York City.

The person she answering said, "All you need to do is get your high school transcript with your IQ scores on it and forward it to us." Therefore, Marie wrote to her high school, got the scores, and sent them to Mensa. Then she waited.

On her next visit to the clinic, Dr. Kruger was sick so Dr. Montgomery took his patients. He was so young Marie immediately questioned his credentials.

"What kind of doctor are you?" She asked as soon as he told her his name.

"I am a psychiatrist. I just graduated last year and I took this job as a way of getting a lot of experience fast."

Marie hoped he could do better than Dr. Kruger, so she started off with a bit of history.

"I was diagnosed with endogenous depression and put on antidepressants. Then my diagnosis was changed to bipolar disorder, and I am now taking lithium."

"That is quite common. The antidepressant throws you into mania, which uncovers your bipolar disorder. Absolutely, you should be taking lithium."

"But I have been taking it for months and it has done me no good. I don't feel any better."

Well, I'm the psychiatrist and I tell you that it is helping and that you just don't know it."

"As the patient, shouldn't I know it?"

"You just may not recognize it. Keep taking it and I promise it will help you."

Marie felt frustrated, alone, and discouraged. She didn't know where to turn. I read the only book in the library about bipolar disorder, and consulted three doctors, she thought. The last two doctors told her that this was the best and only treatment for the disorder, but Marie didn't feel any different. Her mind was still scattered, she still had difficulties, and was confused a lot of the time. It was hard for her to know what to do.

There was something wrong with her, and bipolar disorder, what little she knew about it, explained much of what had gone wrong in her life. She swore she was going to find the answer to this puzzle; and find the solution to this problem.

What would make her "normal" and allow her to manage her relationships and to hang onto her jobs? She, no matter how bad things got, would not apply for disability, which is what the members of the support group had told her to do. Somehow, she would find a way out of this and would take care of herself.

But in her everyday life, it didn't help that some drunk called her regularly on Saturday night at 2 a.m. Her heart jumped into her throat and she answered the phone half-asleep, half-expecting it to be Ted on the line. But it never was.

Every time she went to the clinic, it was the same process: telling the doctor that there had been no change in her mental health, and the doctor insisting that she was better, that she must be better, and that there was no reason why she wouldn't be better. She just didn't recognize how much better she felt. Marie knew this was not true, but no one was listening to her.

After about a month, Marie got a postcard from Mensa headquarters telling her that she qualified for Mensa and giving her the name and number of a guy to call. For the first time in her life, she turned a little shy and it was a few days before she worked up the nerve to call. The guy's name was John and he lived not far from her, in north Oklahoma City.

"John?"

"Yes. "

"I'm Marie. I'm a new member and just got a postcard telling me to call you."

"That's great. Your timing is good. We have a party for new members scheduled here, at my house, on the 17th of next month. Of course, you don't have to wait that long. I can tell you about activities that are happening before then, too."

"No," Marie said. "I think you are right. The timing is too good. I'll wait for the New Member's Party to introduce myself. I'm looking forward to meeting everyone. I'll see you then. Thanks."

Marie was not at all surprised by her eligibility. She was just excited that she had finally made the move and was actually going to be in a position to meet new people after this long period of being almost alone. The next weekend she drove past John's house to be sure of the route, and picked out an outfit well in advance. Marie was ready for something new, hoping that the party lived up to her expectations.

Chapter Twenty-Seven

Marie went to the Mensa New Members' Party after dressing carefully in black pants and a black and gold striped blouse. As she was driving up to the house, she said aloud, "Ted, if you are ever going to come back you better make it soon, because I am going to find someone new tonight."

She arrived exactly on time. She was bad about that; always on punctual for everything, even if you weren't supposed to be prompt at a party. Only about twenty people were there then and Marie talked with most of them. They seemed accepting and asked her questions about her life. One guy was good-looking, with sandy, wavy hair, a chiseled face, and a big smile. He was wearing jeans, a sports jacket and a cowboy hat. His name was Archie.

There was a big keg of beer in the back yard of the house, but since Marie didn't drink that much she didn't indulge. But she loved the fact that all the members came bearing food and the table in the dining room was groaning with what looked like a delicious feast. Finally, one guy came in bearing a roast turkey. Marie sampled most of the goodies and was not disappointed.

By the time the party was in full swing, over one hundred people were there and Marie was a bit dizzy. Almost everyone talked with her, and Archie, who was impossibly good-looking, had asked for her number. He seemed nice. She drove home about one a.m., with Archie following. He insisted on making certain she got home all right.

The next week Marie didn't work every day, and she went to the clinic on Thursday night. Again, she explained to Dr. Kruger that there was no change in her mental functioning, and again he told her she was wrong. He also asked her how she spent her time. She told him about working temporary, and on days she didn't work, she read a book. Dr. Kruger was unbelieving—he said that it was not possible for a person to read a whole book in one day. She told him she had done it her all her life. He didn't seem impressed. He left her with the same prescription; "Take your lithium and you will feel better."

When she got home that night, the phone rang and it was Archie. He asked, "Would you like to go to a Memorial Day picnic with me Saturday around lunch time?"

"Sure, sounds like fun."

Marie couldn't believe someone as cool as Archie asked her out. She really looked forward to the weekend.

On Saturday, Archie picked Marie up and they went to the picnic in the park with a group of Mensans. There were people of all ages there, including a newborn baby. She asked Archie more about his life, and he told her he was divorced, had two children, and worked with computers. She told him about her search for a job, but didn't tell him about her bipolar disorder. She thought it was a little early for that.

As they walked through the park, Archie said, "I carry a knife."

Marie was alarmed. "Whatever for?"

"Oh, in case of emergency."

Marie was getting upset. "What kind of emergency?"

"Something like this." Archie walked out into a field of wildflowers and cut a bunch of them for Marie with his knife. She thought this was the kind of emergency that she could live with.

That night, Archie followed her home and slept on her couch. She didn't know if she was ready for another intimate relationship. When she woke in the morning, he was out on her balcony, cutting muscadine grapes for them to eat at breakfast. He was simply too lovable.

Within a few weeks, they were an item. They usually went to one or two Mensa parties or get-togethers of some sort every weekend. Archie had friends in every group among the many members and Marie met a lot of people and was accepted as Archie's girlfriend.

Marie had forgotten what it was like to be treated as a girlfriend. He took her everywhere, not just to Mensa things but also to his favorite club and to concerts and out to dinner. One night, at the club, one of her Cooper School students, Elizabeth, ran up to her and threw her arms around her. They exchanged greetings and Marie introduced her to Archie. Archie said, "You did have some nice kids at that school, didn't you?"

She hadn't received this treatment in years and thought she had died and gone to heaven. Phideaux joined her in that. He had a man to play with all the time now.

Once he asked her if she thought about getting married. Marie told him that she really had no desire to get married. He seemed a little disappointed, and stated he, at some point, wanted to marry again.

After a while, he told her. "I have this problem. Every few years I get depressed and it lasts for about a year. I won't be able to do anything about it when it happens."

"I understand," Marie said. I am taking antidepressants right now and they have really helped me. The next time your depression hits you, you should try a course of them. They could get you past that."

"I doubt that they would work, but I guess I could try."

"Also, Archie, I need to tell you that I have bipolar disorder and that I am being treated for it. The treatment isn't working. I don't suffer from depression anymore, but I still have ups and downs and can't control my moods."

Archie didn't seem bothered by her admission; he just assumed her problem was a lot like his. It was a good thing she told him, because the next time she went to the clinic, Dr. Kruger told her to try another drug. He said, "Try taking Thorazine at night and see what it does for you."

"I've heard of this. It's supposed to be strong and is used by mental hospitals to keep people under control."

"Pay no attention to what you have heard. Just try it and let me know how it works."

Marie tried a tablet that night at bedtime and the next morning when Archie called, she could barely answer the phone. "Hello?"

"What's wrong with you?" Archie said.

"I—I took a pill. I don't know."

"How many pills did you take?"

"Jus' one."

"I'm coming over there."

A half hour later Marie heard banging on the door and to make it stop, she finally got up and opened the door. It was Archie, who said, "You look awful. Sit on the couch and I'll make you some coffee."

After three cups of coffee, Marie was able to tell Archie what happened. He told her, "Don't ever take that drug again. It's not good for you. I don't want to see you in this shape."

"Okay."

When she went back to the clinic, she told Dr. Kruger, "That Thorazine did not agree with me. I won't take it again."

"It didn't make you feel any better?"

"No, it practically knocked me out cold."

"Well, we'll just continue with the lithium."

"I know," Marie said, "Eventually I'll feel better."

The next week, Marie got good news, at least in some ways. She called Archie to tell him, "I got a job from that interview I had last week."

"Tell me about it."

"It is a social work job that's only a few blocks from my apartment. The job is certifying people for subsidized housing."

"Great," Archie said, "I knew you could do it."

Unfortunately, while the boss did not remember her, they had worked at Child Welfare at the same time and Marie remembered her as not quite right. But hey, it was a job. It paid less than her food stamp job, but certainly better than the temporary jobs, she had been working.

Archie didn't know about the reservations she had. She started work in a week and it was nice to have such a short commute, but the first thing she noticed was that she was the only white person on staff and was immediately excluded socially. Besides her direct boss, Monica, who was a pretty black woman with a short afro, there were three black women on staff. They all did the same thing she did—interview people for Section Eight Housing. It was a lot like Food Stamps but there were no emergencies or duty days. They just took people as their names came up on the lists and interviewed them in turn. They had some troublesome clients but mostly it was routine.

She also had a director who was mostly Native American. Robert was copper-colored red with black hair and bright blue eyes. He was pleasant and really enjoyed his job, and never excluded anyone.

Marie settled in and soon was in a routine. For the first month, everything went along pretty much the same, until one day everyone but Marie went out to lunch—Marie went home for lunch, since she was never invited out with the others, and she lived so close---and when one o'clock rolled around, they didn't come back. A client said, "I have a one o'clock appointment and it is nearly two—when am I going to be seen?"

Marie shrugged her shoulders and said, "I'm sorry, I don't know."

"Where is my worker?"

"I don't know."

Marie was uncomfortable. She had never had this happen in her work life and didn't know what to say or do. She just kept apologizing and wondering to herself where her supervisor and co-workers were. Finally, after two hours, they came in and started seeing their appointments. Marie went to Monica's office and asked her, "What happened?"

"Oh," Monica answered, "We just stopped off after lunch to have our hair done. I think it is one of the perks of the office. You can do it sometime, too."

"Oh, I see." Marie replied. She didn't know what to say or how to react. She had never seen anything so unprofessional in her life. And to leave her alone holding the bag without saying anything to her was appalling. Now Marie didn't feel that she could trust Monica at all.

That evening, while she was still upset over what happened at work that day, Archie called.

"Marie, come over tonight. I'd really like to see you. You can eat dinner with us."

He lived in a large home with a couple, and paid part of his rent by doing handyman work. Marie felt like she really wanted to see him, so she agreed to drive right over.

She got there, parked out front, and simply walked in. They didn't lock the doors when they were home and besides, they were expecting her. She walked all through the house and no one was there. She wondered why he had asked her over and now wasn't home. She couldn't think straight. She drove to a gas station, where she called his number.

She couldn't help it, she was crying when he answered the phone.

"I came over and couldn't find anyone. No one was home. Where were you?"

"We're in the pool. Why didn't you check out back? You should have known we were here. Now come on back. We'll have dinner soon."

Marie felt foolish, and especially since everyone knew about her meltdown. Why did she go off the rails over something that small? She wished she could find the answer to her illness.

Chapter Twenty-Eight

Archie and Marie celebrated their first year together by going to her mother and father's, Peter and Susie's, fiftieth wedding anniversary party. Susie had been looking forward to it eagerly and prepared all the food herself, dips, hors d'oeuvres, cookies, and cakes, an impressive spread.

Aunts and uncles from St. Louis, parts of Texas, and Oklahoma came. There were so many cousins Marie didn't even know how many there were; and all of Pete and Susie's friends were sharing in the party. Susie had a great time and Peter behaved himself. She wore herself out and afterwards Marie and the other kids ordered out for food rather than let her cook the dinner she planned.

One of the funny things about the group was that since they were an Irish family, everyone had greyed early, save one of her young red-haired cousins who stood out in the hall and the dance floor like a beacon.

Marie was happy Archie went with her. All those years with Ted, Marie went to family observances alone. It was nice to have Archie at her side, but Marie was no longer allowed to go over to his place, because the woman he lived with thought she was weird since her meltdown when she thought they weren't home. This made Marie feel her illness had cost her again.

Marie continued to enjoy her membership in Mensa and her relationship with Archie. She also continued going to the Mental Health Clinic, but with the exact same results.

She told her doctor, "I am not any better, but I am determined that I will beat this thing. No matter how hard it is, I am going to continue to work and to support myself."

"You'll lose this job and never work again," Dr. Kruger said, "You are too ill."

"Well, if I will never work, does that mean I will have to go on disability?"

"No, you are not that disabled. You wouldn't qualify."

That confused Marie, but she didn't argue with him, it was too ridiculous. She also didn't change her mind about taking care of herself.

~*~

Archie came by on the weekend as he usually did. "I don't feel like going out tonight. Marie, I told you this would happen. I have started to become depressed and I no longer enjoy doing things. I am going to have to break up with you."

"No, Archie, you said you would try a course of antidepressants if this happened again. Please go to the doctor and ask him for them."

"Okay, I'll try, but I don't think it will do any good."

It didn't seem fair to lose a good relationship because of something she now knew was manageable like depression. She called Archie daily and encouraged him to see the doctor, and reiterated to him how much antidepressants had helped her. Archie didn't feel like coming by to see her, and not only did that make Marie sad, but Phideaux seemed to be depressed, too. He slept all the time, wouldn't eat, and wouldn't play as he usually did.

After a few days Archie reported, "I've been to my doctor and got the prescription, but I am not feeling any better."

"It can take from ten days to two weeks to feel any effect. Please keep trying," Marie said.

"I'll keep trying, meanwhile, I promised to fix your car and I will come by and do that this weekend on Saturday."

On Saturday, Marie was excited, thinking that perhaps Archie would be feeling better and they would patch things up. When he arrived, Phideaux became animated, and kept leaping into the air. Archie said, "I better sit down and make a lap before Phideaux loses it."

He sat down; Phideaux snuggled into his lap and started purring. Marie asked him, "Are you feeling any better?"

"No, I am feeling worse. I just want to get your car fixed so I can go home and stay there. I don't feel like going anywhere or doing anything."

"Archie, I don't know if you realize how sad this makes me. I will really miss you. I love you and depend on you."

"I'm sorry, but there is nothing I can do about it. This is something that has been happening to me all my life. I haven't any control over it."

After Archie finished working on the car, he came in to say goodbye. He hugged Marie and again said, "I'm sorry, I'm not doing this to you on purpose."

Marie cried when he left. Marie hoped to hear from Archie or to run into him at a Mensa function, but she didn't.

At first she thought she wouldn't go back to any Mensa parties, but then realized that she had joined to meet new people would be right back where she started if she let him keep her at home. Marie continued to go to parties by herself not willing to give her Mensa friends up because Archie was ill.

Meanwhile something odd happened while she was distracted by Archie's problems. She began to have symptoms to indicate that she might have cervical cancer. Ignoring it at first, and then remembering what happened to Jackie, she went to her regular GYN. He said, "Take these hormones when you are symptomatic. However, you probably need a hysterectomy and I don't do surgery anymore, so you need to find someone else."

Marie didn't have to think long about this. Eric, her old next-door neighbor, was now a GYN and she trusted him. She made an appointment with him. His assistants and nurse were all bent out of shape when Marie insisted upon calling him "Eric" instead of "Doctor," but they just had to live with it.

Eric did a complete work-up and examination and told Marie, "You have tumors in your uterus."

The next step was a biopsy, which Marie passed, but Eric said, "You still have to have a hysterectomy. What's the insurance situation?"

Marie answered, "I just got this job with the Housing Authority a few months ago. I suppose that this is a pre-existing condition, so I can't have it done right away."

"It should be okay to wait a few months. When do you think you want to do it?"

"How about August? That's the hottest month of the year—I won't mind staying in."

"Okay, we'll tentatively schedule you for August, and I get you set up with the hospital and all."

When Marie went back to work, she told Monica she had to take off in August for surgery. Monica asked her, "Don't you think it would be safer to do it now?"

Marie replied, "Of course I do, but I don't have any way to pay for it right now."

"Well, I would certainly find a way if it were my health problem."

"Monica, I don't have a choice except to wait."

From the way Monica talked about her ex-employees, it seemed to Marie that she always had favorites and always had one person she didn't like. Marie was afraid she was that person now, even though she tried to do the best work she could.

Marie continued to go to Mensa functions and parties, though she often felt out of place by herself. One night she was surprised to find herself interested in a guy she hadn't met before. It turned out that he and his buddy were from Dallas, just up for the weekend. He worked for the FAA and had his own plane. His name was Matt. He was a stocky, balding man who had a great sense of humor and who seemed interested in her, too. That night he had on a baby blue golf shirt and khakis.

He asked her, "Can I call you when I get back to Dallas?"

Marie said, "Of course you can. I would love to talk to you more." She gave him her number and they parted that night with Marie hoping he would call.

Matt called on Monday and they talked for about an hour. He asked her out the next weekend and said he would fly his plane up to see her. She just had to pick him up at the airport.

The "airport" turned out to be a tiny little field whose name she never learned, but she learned how to get there that summer. They started dating and between him flying up to see her and buying tickets for her to fly on Southwest, they saw each other nearly every weekend. On the Fourth, Marie drove to Dallas to spend the weekend with him and on the way back her car broke down. She couldn't get it fixed because of the holiday, so Matt flew up and took her home, then the next weekend, picked her up and took her to get her car.

While they were having a good time with their relationship, Matt said, "Marriage is out of the question for us, because I want to have children."

Marie said, "I understand," but she thought it odd that he was spending time with her since she was not going to be able to have children, and he said he wanted them. She was enjoying herself and wasn't upset that they couldn't get married.

The weekends that she spent in Dallas were fun. He would take her to Mensa functions, and on Sunday mornings, before he flew her back home, they went to the Reunion Tower revolving restaurant for brunch. You could see the whole city from there, and the food was delicious. Matt believed in treating her well.

At work, something weird happened. Monica came to her and said, “Why don’t you use your first name here? You use your middle name instead.”

“Well, no one has ever called me by my first name. I have used my middle name all my life, and that is what I think of as my name.”

Monica answered, “That can’t be true. Your mother must have called you by your first name because otherwise she wouldn’t have named you that.”

“No, my mother named me after my grandmother. At the time, my grandmother lived in our home, and mother didn’t want to have two people in the same house called by the same name, so she used my middle name.”

“I don’t believe that. From now on here, you will be known by your first name, Opal. You don’t have the choice to call yourself any name you want to.”

“But…”

“I told you don’t have a choice. Here we will call you by your proper name.”

It was strange to Marie to be called by a name she had never used, and she didn’t always respond when people at work called her that. She didn’t understand why Monica was so adamant that she use a name she really wasn’t familiar with, and so started looking for another job. But she needed to work here at least until her surgery.

Robert quit without giving a reason. Marie thought she learned why at the next staff meeting. Monica explained her new policy: the workers were to assign white applicants to the projects where mostly white people lived, while the black applicants would go to the projects that had primarily black tenants. Monica said that people would be "more comfortable" with this arrangement.

Marie didn't know what showed on her face, but inside she was frantic. Oh my god, she was saying to herself, at some point, it is going to hit the fan and someone—maybe everyone, is going to be in trouble.

If it hadn't been so close to her operation, Marie would have found a way get out of that job immediately. But it was almost time for her hysterectomy, and if she started over somewhere else, it would start another wait because it was a pre-existing condition. She was on pins and needles but knew she had to stay until after her surgery was done.

Chapter Twenty-Nine

I have you scheduled for eight a.m. on Monday the third. The surgery should be routine, with you leaving the hospital on the fourth or fifth. I propose to recommend that I remove your ovaries because of the history of cancer in your family," Eric, her doctor friend, said.

Marie held up her hand.

"But Eric, I am only forty years old. I'm not at all sure I want that."

"It's no problem. You just take estrogen after your surgery and it'll keep you just as young as your natural hormones."

"I wanted to talk to you about that. For the past two months, I have been having migraine headaches every two weeks. They are awful and last two to three days. The only other time I had a migraine in my whole life was the first month I took birth control pills. They adjusted the dosage and I never had one again. I'm wondering if these hormones I'm taking are causing the headaches."

"No, that's not what's happening. As soon as you have your surgery, your headaches will stop. Trust me on this one. Also, trust me on having your ovaries out. Ovarian cancer is hard to detect and often isn't diagnosed in time. It's best for you to do this."

"All right, if you say so."

At the mental health clinic, Dr. Kruger started raising the dosage of lithium. After a while, Marie's hands started to visibly shake. Marie called the clinic. “Dr. Kruger, my hands are shaking and I am afraid they will see at work.”

“Don’t worry about it. It is a side effect of the lithium, it won’t hurt anything.”

And he raised her dosage again. This time it became difficult for her to write, her hands were shaking so.

Matt called to ask her, “Do you want me to take a week off work and come up to take care of you while you are sick? You know I have never been sick a day in my life, so it would be good experience for me.”

Marie told him. “That is sweet of you, but I have my family here and if you have never been sick you don’t understand how cranky and out of sorts I’m likely to be.”

“But I want to take care of you.”

“I know you do, but believe me, this is better. I’ll call you from the hospital and let you know how I am.”

Marie went into the hospital assuming that she would have a routine surgery and be out in a couple of days. One thing she laughed about to herself was about missing the move. Her parents had their house that they had lived in for over forty years up for sale. The sale went through and they had to move this week. She would be the only one of the five kids not helping.

Eric asked her to bring her lithium to the hospital and medicate herself. He thought that was the easiest way to manage that. She checked in the morning of the operation and had anesthesia at 8 a.m. The surgery seemed to go well and she slept the rest of the day, Friday.

When she woke on Saturday morning, she felt weak and groggy, but assumed that was normal. The staff kept coming in, taking vital signs, taking blood and at first she thought that was normal, too, except it was too often. Then she heard Eric’s voice out in the hall, “You people are practicing some goddamn awful medicine in this hospital.”

That caught Marie's attention, and the young girl who again came in to take her blood was crying. When Eric came in her room, Marie said, "Eric, am I bleeding to death?"

He didn't answer that question.

"We just need a cross-match for a blood transfusion. I ordered it two hours ago and they haven't done it yet."

"But I don't want a blood transfusion. I am too afraid of AIDS."

"Don't worry about that. They have it under control."

"I still don't want one."

"Nevertheless, you are going to have two pints of blood. It's necessary."

"You can't give it to me if I don't want it."

"Yes, I can. You can't get out of that bed. You're too weak."

He demonstrated by using one hand against her chest to hold her in bed.

Afterwards, when she had the transfusions Eric and his resident tried to find out what caused the bleeding. After many tests, they finally discovered that Marie's blood pressure spiked and blew out a blood vessel in her stomach. Everything seemed fine afterwards, but Marie had to spend an extra two days in the hospital. The only good part was that she has to say "No" when the nurse insisted she get up and walk around, because Eric told her not to move around the first two days.

Marie called Matt and told him she would be in the hospital longer. She also told him she was fine and would be going home soon, when she would call him again. Before Eric would discharge her, he made her promise she would pick up a prescription to keep her blood pressure down, because now she had to be on hormones full time and they seemed to affect her blood pressure.

When Marie got home, she wanted to be left alone. Her family was busy, so they just made sure she had medicine and food, and Marie slept. Strange things began to happen.

She started hearing music in her head. It went on nonstop except when she was able to sleep, which wasn't often. She heard "Battle Hymn of the Republic" and the theme of "The Mary Tyler Moore Show" over and over. She had no idea why she was hearing this particular music or why she was hearing music at all. It was most disconcerting—she couldn't read, watch TV, or carry on a conversation and faked it with her family, telling them to just leave her alone, she wanted to rest.

Writing checks with shaky hands was impossible. Her sister Shirley to sign them, knowing the bank no longer looked at signatures. Next, Marie had a meltdown at the pharmacy, where she was well known, because her prescription had run out. The pharmacist was nonplussed; he knew her regular behavior and even renewed her prescription just because he was so worried about her.

Marie called Dr. Kruger and told him what was going on. When he heard all this, he lowered the dosage of her lithium. After a couple of days, to Marie's relief, the music in her head stopped. But Marie really missed Matt, and decided that she wanted to see him. After consulting Eric, she called Matt and asked him to buy her a Southwest Airlines plane ticket for Dallas.

Matt did, and she flew down to spend the weekend with him. However, strange things kept happening. At one point Marie said, "That VW keeps driving up and down the street."

Then Marie started for the door, and Matt said, "Where are you going?"

Marie answered, "I'm going to tell that guy in the VW to stop driving up and down the road."

"No, you aren't. Stay inside."

Later, Matt took her grocery shopping, and then told her to wait while he brought the car up to the door because it was raining. Marie, not paying attention, just got into the first car that drove up. She sat there, looking straight ahead. The car didn't move. She looked around, and the driver was a complete stranger. He was just staring at Marie. She had gotten into the first car that drove up, and it wasn't Matt's car "That was weird," she commented to Matt, when she finally scrambled out of the stranger's car and was in the right one.

He just shook his head. At home, he tried to load the dishwasher, but Marie kept telling him he was doing it wrong and trying to interfere. The weekend was good for Marie, since she was so bored at home, but she thought Matt was glad when she went home at the end of the weekend.

Things started to slow down during her last week at home before she returned to work and she felt more normal. When she returned to work, she felt even more isolated. No one wanted to talk with her or have much interaction with her. She decided to start looking for work elsewhere and just do the job until she could leave. She mentioned to one of the workers that she was going to the doctor that week; she was really referring to her appointment with Dr. Krueger, which was in the evening after work.

Monica called her in and gave her a memo, which stated she had not given Monica notice of her doctor's appointment, so had broken the rules of her employment. She sent the memo to the program director and the vice-president. This upset Marie, who blurted out, "But my doctor's appointment was after work, so it had nothing to do with you. Please send another memo saying that I didn't break any rules."

"No, I won't."

"But I didn't neglect to tell you about the appointment. It wasn't during working hours."

"Well, I have already sent the memo, so it is just too bad."

It was completely unreasonable to Marie, and sounded like she was about to be fired. Marie vowed to be even more careful in the future.

The next week, Marie overheard one of the other workers, Barbara, on the phone with one of her clients.

"Okay, you bring me the twenty dollars and I'll interview you immediately."

Marie really didn't know what to do with this knowledge. Taking bribes was against regulations, but this place was so topsy-turvy she didn't know what was expected of her. After some thought she realized that no matter what the custom of the workplace, the standards were the same everywhere.

She went into Monica's office and told her, "I heard Barbara making a deal with a client to move her up on the waiting list for money."

Monica looked startled and said, "We can't have that. Thank you for telling me."

The next day Marie came into work and Monica told her the vice-president wanted to see her. She went to his office and he told her, right away, she was being "laid off." Marie knew why she was being let go and could have objected or threatened to sue, but she was tired of the place and its values, so she just said "I'm really rather relieved" and left.

It didn't surprise her at all when Matt called a couple of days later and said, "This isn't going to work out for the two of us. I told you that I wanted children and you won't be able to do that. So I think this would be a good time to break it off."

Marie's face squinched up and she started to cry silently. "Okay, Matt, I understand."

She had more or less been expecting it. She knew her behavior at his place was untenable, even though she was unable to control it, and really didn't blame him. However, it made her sad that she had lost another relationship.

Chapter Thirty

You must be psychotic because you had that auditory hallucination." Dr. Kruger said from behind his battered wooden desk at the clinic.

"I don't think I was psychotic, I just overdosed on lithium."

"Anyway, another drug, Haldon, will help you. I need you to sign a release before I can give it to you, though."

This release stated she knew about the side effect known as tardive dyskinesia. Marie knew about it all right, and had seen some patients with it. It is involuntary, constant movements of the face or mouth. If she developed it, she would never find another job.

"I am not going to sign the release because I am not willing to risk getting tardive dyskinesia."

Dr. Kruger laughed at her, saying, "It is only a problem with older people, people in their sixties. You don't have to worry about it."

"Okay, in that case I'll sign, if you really think the new drug will help.

Marie signed the release, and Dr. Kruger prescribed the Haldon. Marie took it but, again, it didn't seem to improve her mental status, to stop her mood fluctuation or make her stop being so irritable.

Despite that, Marie applied for unemployment and started looking for work again. She was happy to be done with the Housing Authority, but scared about her future. There was nothing she hated more than looking for work; it may not have been the best idea to get a history degree. Great time to decide that, she thought.

This time she came across a temporary job that sounded interesting and paid well for a temp job. It was a job "digesting depositions." That simply meant summarizing the information in depositions in a large legal case so the attorneys could access it easier. Marie applied for the job and got it. She found that she really had a talent for it and it was easy work. The hard part was sitting still for hours when she was still somewhat manic.

Every two weekends, she had a migraine. It didn't mean that she had to miss work, but it ruined her whole weekend and meant that she couldn't go to Mensa activities. If she had promised to do something at Mensa, she had to back out. It really upset her when she had to break her word.

She worked at the job for months. Since Marie was such a fast reader and good with summarizing, she was able to do twice the volume of work as anyone else. However, she was manic most of the time and was irritating to the other employees, talking too much, too fast and always right there with an opinion. She was not really aware of this, though.

The lithium she was taking was not working, and the antidepressant was not being buffered by any other medication, so she stayed manic most of the time. This did not help her relationships, whether romantic or friendships.

After Marie worked there for six months, she was eligible for a raise. That same week, the supervisor announced, "Anyone who misses work for any reason will be fired."

The raise would have kicked in on Monday, but Marie's migraine came early that week, on Friday afternoon. She was not able to work with a blinding headache and upset stomach, so she went home. The lead worker called her at home, "You've been fired for leaving work."

"But I had a migraine. I couldn't sit there and read and write with a headache like that.

"Sorry, we don't accept any excuses."

So it was back on unemployment, which lasted only a few weeks more. Marie went back into teaching part time at local junior colleges. She was assigned two classes, but the pay was so low, only a thousand dollars per course, it really was not enough to live on.

She had always wanted to teach, and this was a perfect opportunity to try it again. To her distress, she found that her inability to concentrate and her (what she later recognized as manic behavior) made her a less than mediocre teacher. She had spent years in school assuming that she would be a great teacher, and now she recognized that she was not doing a good job. But she continued, needing the money.

It did give her enough time to go to the University Hospital to try to find out why she was having these migraines. She suspected the hormone replacement therapy, but Eric told her that was ridiculous. She had no insurance, and when she tried to go to a private doctor to be diagnosed, the doctor told her to go to the University hospital "where she belonged" and then charged her fifty dollars for that piece of advice.

After waiting all day at University Hospital, Marie finally got an appointment with a neurologist. When she returned for the appointment, he, who was actually a resident, looked at her record and said,

"You are mentally ill. You aren't having migraine headaches; you are only imagining that you are."

"But Doctor, I need some kind of pain management. These headaches are a killer."

"No, pain pills won't help. You aren't really having headaches so there is nothing I can do."

Every doctor she consulted told her: “The hormones are vital to your health and you need to keep taking them. There is no way they can cause headaches.”

“But it says on the package insert that they may cause migraines.”

“That is really, really rare. It couldn’t be true in your case.”

Meanwhile, Marie’s blood pressure went sky-high and so did her cholesterol level. When she pointed out these sudden spikes, doctors told her, “It is due to ‘old age’.”

They gave her cholesterol and blood pressure medication.

At Mensa, she met and started dating Jacob. Without even consulting her, he moved in after ten days. At first, they got along quite well, but after a few weeks they started to argue. Jacob was buying the groceries, while Marie paid the rent. Jacob didn’t like Marie’s diet, and refused to buy, for example, the cereal she liked.

“There are cheaper cereals you can eat and I’ll only buy those. Also, I know you love rice but you are eating white rice and you should be eating brown rice. It is better for you.”

“I’m sure it is, but I don’t like brown rice, and I won’t eat it.”

“That’s the only kind I will buy you.”

Marie sat him down and told him, carefully and slowly, “Jacob, I am forty-two years old and you cannot tell me what to eat. I am a grown woman, not a child, and I get to choose what I eat.”

“Oh, I understand that,” he said, “No problem.”

Then he continued with the same behavior, just as if she had never talked with him about it.

When it came to politics, they could not agree. Jacob was one-sixteenth Native American. He told Marie, “That is my identity.”

Marie retorted, “But you have blond hair and blue eyes.”

"That doesn't matter, I am still a Native American, and it is people like your grandmother who took part in the Cherokee Strip Land Run who took my land away from me."

"What would you have me do about it? She lost the land the second year because of a drought."

"It's the principle of the thing."

He insisted that all politics were racial. One example was; "The atomic bomb was developed to be used on Japan and it was never intended to be used on Germany."

As a history major, Marie disputed that. "The bomb was being developed with the fear that the Nazis would get it first, but it was not ready to be tested until July 17, after VE day, so it couldn't be used on Germany."

Jacob just looked at her. Nothing Marie ever said made him think about his opinion on anything. It was like talking to the wall.

Marie made the comment, while reading some of his works, that Churchill was the greatest writer of English she had ever read. Jacob became angry, because Churchill was a "colonist." He argued it was "well-known" that Leslie Charteris, who wrote "The Saint" was the most talented writer of English, ever. It was almost impossible to hold a conversation with him: Marie buried her head in her hands. She didn't even point out it was Churchill who won the Nobel Prize in literature.

For the first time in her life, Marie found herself financially dependent on a man. She couldn't break up with him because she couldn't support herself. She was at a loss. Her unemployment had run out, she made only a pittance teaching, she didn't know how she could work due to her headaches, or live eating brown rice.

Marie decided to stop taking hormones on her own, after a particularly bad weekend and the migraines stopped immediately. Her blood pressure dropped back to normal.

Okay, maybe she was supposed to take hormones, but she couldn't face the side effects anymore. So for now, she was off them.

The next time she went back to Dr. Kruger, he asked her how the new drug was working. Marie told him that it seemed to have no effect on her. He acted as though he didn't believe her, but gave her another drug, Navane.

Twice, Marie had to pay the rent for her apartment with her credit card. She kept thinking that something would come through for her, but nothing did. She couldn't keep up with her payments on her credit card and she lost it. Then she had incessant calls from bill collectors, which she had never experienced before. She would curse them out because she was so frustrated. Eventually, they left her alone.

She was wondering why she couldn't get any traction when she saw an ad while watching TV that gave her hope.

The ad was for continuing education, and mentioned paralegal education. Wow, Marie thought that would be just right for me. Immediately, she picked up the yellow pages and found the schools in town. There was the one she was once Registrar of, and then another. She knew the quality of the one she worked at, so she checked into the other one and found that it had a good reputation.

She had an appointment with Dr. Kruger, so she went in to talk with him and the social worker. Dr. Kruger was not in, so she was interviewed by another doctor. He said, "Are you hearing voices or seeing things?"

"No, several months ago I heard music," and she explained about the auditory hallucination.

The doctor said, "You are often more manic right after you have anesthetic. That was probably it. You shouldn't be taking Navane, especially since you say it is not doing any good. It is likely to cause tardive dyskinesia."

"But I was told that would only happen to people in their sixties, and I'm in my forties."

"No, you are quite vulnerable to it at your age. I recommend you discontinue it."

Marie decided to stop taking the drug as the doctor recommended, but she also wanted to speak to the social worker. She stopped by her office and saw the social worker was alone, so she didn't have to wait in line.

"Is there any financial help for me to go to school?" Marie asked.

The social worker looked up and said, "No, no help for you."

Marie found that discouraging, but she wasn't going to give up that easily.

The next day she took her college transcript and signed up with the school she wanted to attend. She was admitted, and signed papers for a $5,000 student loan. She knew she would have to pay it off, but she would have a job! No problem.

A few days later Jacob started in with one of his off-the-wall theories, and Marie turned to him and said, "Why don't you get your shit and get out of my house?"

After he was gone, she realized it was the first break-up she had gone through with no regrets.

Chapter Thirty-One

With her hopes up, Marie started paralegal school, located in a strip mall not far from her apartment. The thirty-five women in her class were younger and more affluent than Marie, but they seemed nice enough.

One student said, "I can't wait to get into these classes. I think this is the kind of career I can really enjoy." That seemed to the consensus of thought among all the students.

The classes were taught by local lawyers and paralegals covered all aspects of law and the functions of a paralegal. Marie found herself asking numerous questions and interrupting the speaker constantly. She couldn't help it. She could see the dirty looks she was getting, but just kept doing it.

School was a fulltime job. Classes lasted from nine in the morning until three in the afternoon plus hours of homework each night. Some of the students seemed to struggle. One told her, "I can't believe they are serious. This is more work that anyone could do."

Marie answered, "No, it isn't. You just have never been to graduate school. It's not as hard as getting an M.A."

That girl seemed to think Marie was bragging and wouldn't have anything to do with her after that. Marie felt bad because she didn't have decent clothes to wear. She kept gaining weight on the drugs they gave her at the clinic and finally totaled one hundred and sixty pounds. She didn't even recognize herself.

One lunch hour she dashed downtown to pick up her meds at the clinic. Considering her busy day ahead of her, it would be best to get chore out of the way. She drove as fast as she dared, raced into the clinic and stood in line behind one other person. The clerk finished, at about a minute to noon. Marie only needed a paper from her to take to the pharmacist, who stayed open during lunch.

The clerk reached up to pull her window "Closed" and Marie said, "Oh, please, don't close up, this will only take a minute."

The clerk said, "Too bad," and closed her window.

Marie almost cried, it was so frustrating. She went back to school and finished out the afternoon, then made another run to the clinic in a lot more traffic than before and stood in a much longer line to get her paper that would allow her to get her meds.

She happened to run into the Director of the clinic and took that opportunity to complain about the clerk, who had refused to wait on her that morning. "I was here just about a minute or two minutes before noon and she closed up in my face, forcing me to make another trip here. Now it is hard going to school fulltime, with so little money, and you're making my life more difficult rather than helping."

"You're going to school? Why aren't you getting Rehabilitation funding?"

"I asked the social worker if there was any help for me to go to school, and she said there wasn't, so I took out a student loan."

"I'll have to talk with her. You should have received total funding to go to school. And I will speak to the clerk about being more sensitive to client's needs."

"Thanks," Marie said," I appreciate that."

That night, while she was working on a paper for school, she got a phone call. "Hello?"

"Hello, I'm the social worker from the Mental Health Clinic."

"Yes?" said Marie.

"The Director spoke to me today about you going to school and not getting Rehabilitation funds. I just checked my records and they show I set up a meeting with you to discuss funding for your schooling, but you said you didn't want to come to the meeting."

"No, that's not what happened. I asked you for help and you said there wasn't any."

"Well, the fact I set up a meeting with you and that you refused to come to is right here in my records in black and white."

"Oh, I see. Well, I hope you are happy with that."

"Good-bye."

Marie put her head in her hands and cried a little. She knew there was no fighting that one. She should have pushed harder when she asked for help, and requested a supervisor. Instead, she just accepted what the social worker said without questioning it.

She was the crazy one and the social worker was just named "Social Worker of the Year" at the clinic. Again, she had been too trusting and this time she lost five thousand dollars. She vowed to use a tape recorder in any future transactions like that one. It was so maddening. She couldn't afford to get a private doctor to help her with her bipolar disorder, but she couldn't seem to get any help from the mental health clinic. She was trying so hard to get through school and to find the right medication for her illness, but no one seemed ready to help her.

School lasted four months, and Marie was glad she had learned not to procrastinate in graduate school. She had one friend, Jerri, who sat beside her and talked with her every day. Jerri had a big house and a demanding husband, and she surprised Marie by asking, "Marie, will you help me clean my house on Friday afternoons? I'll pay you thirty-five dollars a week."

Marie started that week. The house was a condo next to a pond with six other condos built around it. The pond had swans on it and was lovely. The condos were expensive and had all the latest appliances, including a vacuum cleaner built into the walls and huge bathrooms with enormous mirrors. Jerri said, "My husband insists that the house be spotless for the weekend, so I can really use your help."

Marie could see why she needed help with such a big house. Jerri was nice and fun to work with and Marie gained a little more income.

The school term passed quickly. There was so much to do, and so much to learn that graduation in December came faster than it seemed possible. Marie started looking for a job right away, purchasing a new suit for job interviews. She did get some interviews, but no jobs. Marie didn't realize how much she had tried the patience of her classmates until she met a woman who she sat behind in the class. They ran into each other downtown and Marie started to speak with her, but realized that the person was not even going to acknowledge her. That really hurt.

One of the paralegals at the school advised the graduates, "Be sure and check with all the temporary paralegal agencies. There are tons of temp jobs out there."

Marie applied with several of them, and got some assignments. Most of the jobs were boring filing jobs, but they paid ten dollars an hour because they were paying for training and confidentiality. This made it a lot easier to pay the bills.

Then she saw that her old job as a deposition digester was open. She didn't have migraines anymore, plus now she had a paralegal certificate. If they had a big case, she might be able to get some steady income. So she went to their office to apply.

While she was waiting to interview, she spoke up and told the guy next to her, "I used to work here, but just a day before I was supposed to get a raise, I was fired. Other than that, it is a good place to work."

Marie knew the woman, Pam, who interviewed her and told her how she had gotten rid of her migraines, and had also been to paralegal school. "I know that I did a good job for you last time and I would be even more valuable to you now."

"You are right, you did a good job last time we set up shop here and we could use your experience. We'll hire you back starting Monday at the rate you were making when you left."

"Thank you," Marie said, "I'll see you on Monday."

About an hour after she got home, Pam called her. "You know what? Right after I interviewed you, I talked with a man who told me about a woman who said that she used to work for us but we fired her just before she was to get a raise. Now I can't think of anyone else but you who would say such a thing who was in today. Don't bother to come in Monday."

Marie said, "But I would still do a good job for you."

"Good-bye."

Marie was shaken, and she questioned her judgment. How could she have been so stupid? That job would have guaranteed her a steady income while she looked for a better job, and she had opened her big mouth for no good reason. She couldn't blame anyone but herself for losing that job.

Chapter Thirty-Two

Marie's temporary assignments got farther apart and shorter in duration. She didn't know if she was displeasing the bosses or if she was getting bad references from the students she was in school with, but somehow her work was diminishing

She had little income and the only thing that saved her was that Uncle Paul died and left her a few thousand dollars. Her mother was upset about Paul's death; she had been like a mother to all her younger brothers. Marie had never been too fond of him, but was sorry it made her mother feel bad. She would have liked to spend the money on a nice vacation or a down payment on a new car, but instead she used it to pay her student loan and her rent.

Gas was so expensive that going to Mensa activities was out of the question. She was also losing her classes at the Junior Colleges because the department heads weren't happy with her teaching. She wasn't preparing her classes well and her casual delivery of information upset some of the students, though others liked it. She was down to one class a semester.

Marie did something so weird at the grocery store that she couldn't even believe it herself. This was the store she frequented weekly, and was well known there. While looking around, she spied some eye shadow that was pretty. She couldn't spend money for something like that—all she could buy at that time were the essentials. But she really wanted that eye shadow.

Before she knew what happened, her hand snaked out and she snared it and slipped it into her pocket. Nobody said anything to her, so she assumed she got away with it. Later, she thought they could have seen her and did not want to deal with it. She didn't know, but for weeks, she was amazed at herself for doing such a thing. It didn't keep her from using the eye shadow.

By the time Marie was out of school six months, she was desperate. Nothing was going well, and she felt as she did back in Norman five years ago. There she had turned to the mental health center for help. This time the mental health center wasn't the answer. She thought the only thing to do was to go to a hospital where she would get a complete work-up and more attention. On her next visit to the center, she asked the doctor about going to the hospital.

"Are you suicidal?" he asked.

"No, I am not suicidal, I am homicidal!" Marie said emphatically. "I don't know what to do or where to turn. I am angry and don't know what to do with my anger. I want some kind of solution. My life hasn't improved in the years I've been coming to this clinic. It's been five years and I'm in the same shape I was when I came here. I'm not getting any better.

No one seems interested in helping me. No one listens to me when I say that I am not getting any better. There has to be a way for me to get better, to get some treatment that will really help. I am tired of taking drugs that don't work and my life not improving at all. I am wasting my time here."

"I can get you into the State Mental Hospital, but you know the minimum stay is six weeks, so you would probably lose your apartment."

"What about my cats?" Marie asked.

"Give them away."

"No, I have to find some other solution. This won't work for me. Besides, I don't believe the treatment at the State Hospital would be any different than what I am getting here."

Marie wanted something different, something that would work, and she didn't trust the system she had been involved with for the past five years to suddenly come up with something that would work for her. She felt like she was on her own and was responsible for her own care.

Well, she had always been on her own, she thought, so she might as well take care of this, too.

Somehow, Marie got it in her head that private mental hospitals had to have, by law, a bed or beds for public patients. She didn't know how she got that idea, but decided to try to find a place for herself without involving the clinic.

She sat down with the telephone book and started calling all the private mental hospitals in town. "Hello, I understand that you have one or a number of free beds for the public in your hospital. Is this correct?"

"No, this is a private hospital. We don't have any free beds."

None of the people who answered the phones at the hospitals knew what Marie was talking about. After ten or fifteen calls, she got so frustrated she blurted out, "Well, if I can't get any help, I guess I'll just have to kill myself!" Marie really felt at that time if she didn't get any help she would have to commit suicide. Her life was not worth living unless she got some help with her medication and her illness.

Scared, the operator called the Oklahoma City Police Department, and two patrolmen came to Marie's apartment in no time to see if she was all right The cops were young, Boy Scout-types, concerned about Marie, and a little shaky on the concept of mental illness. One of them said, "Now don't you be taking any of those pills—they'll make you crazy." She explained to them that she needed to go to a hospital but didn't want to go to the state hospital because she wanted different treatment from what she had been receiving at the mental health clinic. They knew something that was a tremendous help to Marie.

One of them said to her, “If you want to go to a hospital, you know where you ought to go? There is a clinic at University Hospital that specializes in your kind of problem. It’s on the Ninth Floor of the hospital. They’ll have you in and out in no time. Just tell them that Officer Thompson referred you.”

“That’s all I have to do? Just show up and give them your name?”

“That’s it. I’ll call them and tell them you are coming. Good luck.”

University Hospital was a teaching hospital, working with the medical students of the University of Oklahoma. Marie didn’t know about the clinic, and she didn’t know how to get referred there, even though she was an ex-social worker and had been diagnosed for five years with bipolar disorder. There was no set period of time you had to stay and it specialized in mood disorders. It sounded exactly like what she needed.

Marie called two of her friends at the apartment complex and when they got to her place, said "Can you take care of my cats for a while?”

They spoke almost at once. “Why, is something wrong?” “Are you going somewhere?”

“I’ve told both of you that I have bipolar disorder and that I am not getting any help from the mental health clinic. Well, I lost it a couple of hours ago when it looked like I wouldn’t ever get any help I blew up and somebody called the police and they came out. They referred me to a clinic at University.”

Christy spoke up, “That sounds like a great idea.”

“University is a good hospital. I’ll bet they can help you.”

“What I need from you two is for you to take care of Phideaux and Peave while I am gone. I don’t know how long I will be there, but I will buy plenty of food and they know you and trust you. I would appreciate it so much.” Marie held out her hands in appeal.

“You took care of my cats last summer when we were on vacation, so I will be happy to help you out,” Christy said.

Sherry was a little dubious, but said. “You know I’ve never had a cat but yours are special. They come to see me every day when I come home from work. If you’ll show me what to do, I’ll take my turn, with Christy backing me up.”

“Thank you both so much. Now I can go into the hospital without worrying about them. That makes it so much easier. I really appreciate it.”

I know you both work during the day and I don’t want you to spend your time visiting me. You’ll be doing enough by caring for the cats. That is such a help for me I can’t tell you how much it will help me. I’m leaving this evening, so I have made a key for each of you. I swear, this time I am going to come back sane!” They all laughed at that.

Chapter Thirty-Three

That evening found Marie standing outside the locked doors of the Ninth Floor of University Hospital perusing the papers she had to sign to be admitted. Never having been in a mental hospital before, she had no idea what to expect. The first thing a person had to do was to sign herself in as a suspected crazy person. The papers surprised Marie—she was signing herself in voluntarily, but when she wanted to leave, the doctors had three days to decide whether she would be allowed to do so. That was not what she expected; Marie thought she could leave at any time by just signing herself out. But desperate times call for desperate measures, so she signed the papers and then was admitted, nervous and unsure, her insides churned with anxiety.

The nurse who let Marie into the locked ward took her to what looked like a dorm room. "This will be your room while you are here. You are responsible for keeping it neat and for making the bed. I need to take your shampoo and conditioner and other personal care products, your razor and any mirrors you might have." Marie opened her suitcase and surrendered the items the nurse asked for.

Marie didn't like losing her personal belongings, but she was willing to try almost anything to get better. It seemed like a violation of her privacy, worse than being back in college when the nuns always wanted to know what was going on with her life.

When Marie saw the young residents and interns scurrying around the ward, she realized that she just did something she always been advised not to. She checked herself into a teaching hospital at the end of June just before the new crop of interns and residents came on board. Well, it was too late for regrets now. She was going to be training doctors and getting what she needed was all up to the luck of the draw.

Marie constantly wondered if she had made a mistake, but was determined to see this through. The nurses were predominately middle-aged psychiatric nurses. It looked like some of them knew what was going on. She didn't see an option, so she resolved to take things calmly. She was hyper-alert, though.

Before joining the patient population, a nurse briefed on her on the rules.

"Smoking is allowed on this ward only," she said, "because it is so difficult for people with mood disorders to quit smoking. You are expected to take part in all activities, and to ask permission before doing anything."

Marie was grateful to hear the smoking rule. Smoking was not allowed in any other part of the hospital, and she had been worried about that. The idea of quitting smoking and getting better at the same time seemed overwhelming.

"Since it is a teaching situation," the nurse said, you will be undergoing testing for just about everything—and you will cooperate with all the tests. The doors to the ward are locked at all times, and patients checked on at night every quarter-hour. You are not to be in your room alone except to be in the bathroom."

Since Marie was rather a loner and liked to spend part of every day reading, this was starting to sound difficult. But she wanted treatment more than anything, so she agreed. Actually, she didn't think she had a choice but to agree.

That evening, Marie participated in a long interview with a psychiatric nurse. She asked, "Can you give me a medical history?"

"Where should I start?" asked Marie.

"We'll need childhood diseases, any hospital stays, and surgeries."

"Let's see, I had a tonsillectomy in 1947, and I've had the usual: whooping cough, mumps, measles, and chicken pox. She continued describing illnesses and hospitalizations right up until her hysterectomy; after that, the nurse asked for her mental health history.

"I tried counseling about seven years ago. Diagnosed with depression, and told simply that 'I should get over it.' I didn't get much out of that. Then, five years ago, the Mental Health center in Norman diagnosed me with endogenous depression and gave me an antidepressant. That uncovered my bipolar disorder, and since then I've been going to the Mental Health center here in the City, taking lithium and some anti-psychotics, but nothing has helped so far."

The nurse asked for a social history, and was disbelieving when Marie told her she worked at twenty-seven jobs in the last three years. It did sound a little unlikely, but it was the truth. Every time Marie lost a job, she had to go out and get another one right away.

After this, Marie's intern asked for the same information. Marie patiently recited it for him, willing to put up with it if it was to result in some help. Following the interviews, Marie met her roommate who was depressed, but had been put on antidepressants and almost ready to go home.

Marie asked for shampoo and conditioner so she could get ready for bed. She decided the shampoo thing was simply a control measure—Who ever heard of suicide by shampoo? Of course, an attempt could be rather messy, so maybe that was the reason for the rule.

The patients were expected to take part in various activities during the day—exercise, art projects, group therapy, and other undertakings. After dinner, the TV was turned on and they were allowed to watch "Wheel of Fortune." Marie's claim to fame was that she was acknowledged as the best player on the ward. They also played scrabble and other board games. Most people had visitors during these hours but Marie, embarrassed, asked people not to visit her.

All night long that first night, the bedroom door opened and the nurse flashed a light around to make sure the patients weren't doing anything forbidden, like killing themselves. It was distracting, but soon Marie was used to it and learned to sleep right through the bed checks.

The next morning, she had to obtain her mirror and sat on the floor in the hall to put on her make-up. They had to do it in public so they couldn't break a mirror and hurt themselves. However, if they wanted to shave their legs, or when the men shaved, they checked out a razor and shaved in private. It was all strange and somewhat absurd. Marie stopped asking questions. She was always told, "It's just the rules."

That day they scheduled each of them for batteries of tests, more for the benefit of the interns and residents than for the patients. There were several tests; two of them were an EEG and a brain scan, for example.

Marie met her resident that day. Dr. Jim Schaefer. He listened patiently to her list of the medications she had taken, none of which had seemed to do any good for her manic-depression. Dr. Schaefer was a man of few words and after Marie's monologue, he simply said, "Well, I guess we won't give you lithium."

For the first time Marie felt that someone had heard her. He said, "I'm going to prescribe Tegretol, which is an anti-seizure medication. For some reason, this type of medication works when lithium doesn't. No one knows why. You can start it as soon as the lithium is out of your system."

Finally, she was hopeful something positive would from of the experience.

After this, Marie met the other patients. There were sixteen of them, counting Marie—mostly mood disorders, which were primarily depressed and bipolar patients. But there was also a patient with obsessive-compulsive disorder, a young girl with schizoid personality disorder, a young boy with mild schizophrenia, and even a patient with multiple personality disorder. Between activities, during smoke breaks (and they all smoked), they told each other their stories.

A young, good-looking kid, named Tim, was getting out in a couple of days. He was so pleased and confided in her, "I was taking drugs and my father kicked me out of the house. I moved in with a friend, and his mother asked me why I took drugs. I told her that it was just to shut up the voices in my head. She told me 'you're not supposed to have voices in your head' and she looked for a place to help me. I had just turned eighteen and was able to sign myself into University when she found this clinic. The doctor gave me a minimal dose of Haldon and the voices have gone away. I feel peaceful for the first time in years."

Marie spoke up, "But you know you can't take drugs anymore?"

"The doctor explained that I can't take street drugs at all and that I have to take Haldon from now on. Right now, I just can't wait to get out of the hospital and get on with my life. My friend's mother has explained everything to my parents, and I am going home. I also have several girlfriends waiting for me."

Middle-aged Jean was obsessive-compulsive, and couldn't make her visions go away. "The visions intrude on my life and make it hard for me to function." Marie asked her what they were like and she said, “They are scenes from American life like I have seen in history books.”

Marie wanted to laugh, it sounded so ridiculous, but it was obvious they upset Jean and had landed her in a mental health hospital. Marie sympathized with her and asked her about her treatment.

Jean said, “The doctor gave me this rubber band to wear on my wrist and I am supposed to pop myself whenever I have a vision. This should stop them.”

Marie remembered how much good the antidepressants had done her, and thought she would have asked for medication if it were her. But she didn’t say anything to Jean; it wasn’t Marie’s business.

The young girl, Margie, was a “cutter,” a person who cut herself compulsively with a razor blade. She didn’t know why she did it or how to stop it. Marie never learned her treatment, or how successful it was, since Margie remained hospitalized after she left.

The girl with multiple personality disorder stayed completely away from the rest of the patients, and seemed to be there just so the doctors could learn about her. She was always on suicide watch, and Marie and the others learned nothing about her or her treatment.

Marie and the other patients were allowed to stay up late on the Fourth of July. They sat in the windows of the hospital, watching the various fireworks displays though out the City. It was probably the best view in the City but it wasn’t very festive. Marie sadly had to watch the festivities from her perch in the window of the nuthouse, but her sadness was tempered by the hope that she would soon be able to manage her life better.

Chapter Thirty-Four

Some of the patients liked being in the hospital. They had no responsibilities, their food was provided for them, their lives scheduled, and they made no decisions. Marie hated it, hated having to ask for her own possessions, hated being scheduled, and purely hated being locked up. Just the idea of being locked up, of not being able to leave, even though she wanted to be there, tormented her.

For example, a former patient who had once been on the ward missed the daily paper during his stay and now paid for a subscription for the patients. Every day, they read the newspaper, except for the day it didn't come. Marie asked an intern, "If I give you a quarter, will you go out and get me a newspaper?"

"Sorry, don't have time," he replied.

Then she asked a nurse, "Will you let me out the door just long enough to buy a paper from the vending machine that's just outside the door?"

"No, I'm sorry, I can't do that." Little things like that were so frustrating.

When it came time for Marie's roommate to be discharged, she cried. "I just can't make it out there."

Marie asked her, "Can you make supper for your boyfriend?"

She said, "Yes."

Marie said, "Can you go to the grocery store and buy food?"

She said, "Yes."

Marie said, "Can you keep the house clean?"

She said, "Yes."

Marie then said, "Well, you don't have to be President of the United States, you just have to be able to handle those sorts of things." She immediately brightened up and packed to go home.

After a few days, Marie was able to try the medication Dr. Schaefer prescribed for her, Tegretol, and within a week, she was improving. She was stabilizing and soon felt better than she ever had. Marie was able to take things in stride and felt more in control of herself than ever before. Her thoughts came more slowly and weren't so fractured. She had a better handle on her moods, which didn't fluctuate gratuitously. Marie felt like Dr. Schaefer had given her the key to let her out of hell. She didn't think about suicide, or babble on uncontrollably. She felt "normal."

Dr. Schaefer agreed that the drug was working and it seemed to be the solution for her. However, Marie asked him, since she was in the hospital already, if he would try her on another hormone replacement therapy. Unfortunately, this regimen made her even sicker than previous one she tried. Her blood pressure shot up to two hundred over one-fifty and not only did it cause a migraine, but she also threw up constantly.

This meant that Marie couldn't leave the hospital until the drugs were out of her system. But she was happier than ever, and felt that she could handle her life for the first time. She asked her intern, "Can I lose all this weight I gained on lithium and antidepressants now?"

He said, "There is no reason why you can't. Tegretol doesn't make you gain weight."

Marie vowed to go on a diet as soon as she was released from the hospital. The weight gain was one of the things that made her so unhappy about her diagnosis. She knew dieting wouldn't be easy, but at least know it was possible.

Dr. Schaefer asked, "Marie, please make arrangements for your parents to talk with me. I think I need their input."

They came to the interview, but neither the doctor nor the parents ever told Marie what was said. They also never asked her why she was in a locked hospital ward or what went on there. It was as if it never even happened.

Marie became anxious, and began to think of Ted. She finally realized that all that behavior she thought was strange was actually Ted acting out his bipolar disorder. His drinking, his drug taking, his cyclic disappearances all added up to a case just like hers. No wonder they couldn't get along!

Marie was upset she confided in one of the nurses and the nurse asked what she was going to do about it. Marie said, "I want to write him a letter so it will at least be in his head that there is a possibility that he has bipolar disorder if he ever needs help."

The nurse thought that was a good idea, if not for Ted's sake, but to make Marie feel better.

Marie composed a letter and sent it to the only address she could think of, a professional journalism group Ted belonged to. Of course, she never heard back from him, but she felt that she had done as much as she could to help him.

Marie made friends with a middle-aged man, Bob, who was depressed and an alcoholic. To add to his problems, his wife decided to leave him while he was in the hospital. Marie felt sorry for him and wanted to help him keep his mind off his troubles. Marie and Bob spent time together on breaks, worked the newspaper's crossword puzzle together each morning, and teased each other. Bob would say, "Hey, I'm going to sneak into your room tonight and freak the nurse out when she comes for bed check."

The nurses kept a close eye on them because they really were afraid they were starting an “inappropriate relationship.” One thing he did do for Marie was inappropriate—She had a pair of scrubs that were comfortable and decent for her to wear considering her increase in weight, but the elastic at the waist broke and she had to walk around holding them up. The nurses would not give Marie a safety pin for fear she would hurt herself with it, but Bob smuggled one in to her after his weekend leave. It was most appreciated.

Marie wasn’t allowed weekend leaves because her migraines kept her from some of the activities and she had been dubbed “uncooperative.” Jean got angry at this, and said about the migraine, “but you were sick as a dog!” Marie didn’t try to fight it, because she knew that “rules are rules” and they wouldn’t make an exception because she was sick. It would make the other patients think they could skip activities and get away with it. Marie could hear them saying it.

Bob was a MASH sergeant in the Army, and the ward was right next to the helipad where helicopters landed with emergencies. One of the patients’ major diversions was watching them land. Marie asked Bob why they were so slow and deliberate with the patients, while in the TV show “MASH” they always grabbed the stretchers and ran with them. He laughed, and explained that in those cases there were usually one or more helicopters above waiting to land. “Oh,” Marie replied, feeling somewhat dumb.

At his request, Marie went to an AA meeting with him, and found that she did not like the touchy-feely atmosphere of the meeting. He needed her moral support, though, and she attended when he wanted her to and when her schedule allowed.

Marie also went to a bipolar support group in the hospital, which could have been helpful, but wasn’t. Marie had problems with herself. She was sure now that medication stabilized her that she didn't need anything else. She wanted to live her life as if she didn't have an illness. She told herself she wasn't like those people in the support group; she had it all together and didn't need their help. Marie was certain she was stable for life and wouldn't need any more help than her medication. All she had to do was to take it and she would be fine. She didn't need no stinkin' support.

The ward had a blood pressure monitor on a little cart, which creaked as it was pulled along. Every hour one of the nurse's aides took Marie's blood pressure, monitoring it often because it was so high. The others teased her about it, laughingly saying, "Marie, they're coming for you" when they heard the creaking start from across the building.

Marie's blood pressure finally began to go down and it was looking as if she was going to get out. Since she didn't have any income at all, a social worker visited her on the ward and assured her that the county would pay her hospital bill. With that out of the way, Marie called her mother and asked her to pay her rent on her apartment for the next month, which she promised to do. These two things made her biggest worries disappear.

Before she left, Marie met Michael, who had just checked in. He was more of a "classic" manic-depressive. Michael was horribly depressed, thin, with unkempt hair. He lay in a fetal position on a bench, explaining, "This has happened to me before. All I need is some lithium and I'll be all right." Marie worried about him; he looked so thin and pitiful.

That was his condition when Marie left the hospital, so she didn't even recognize him when she ran into him at a luncheonette downtown a couple of months later. He was dressed in a suit, confident-looking with a sharp haircut and when he said, "Hello, how are you?"

Marie had to say, "I know I know you, but could you tell me where we met?"

Mike laughed and said, "Don't you remember, Marie? We were both patients at University Hospital."

Marie smiled. "I guess the lithium did it for you."

He said, "Oh, yes, it always works." Marie asked him how much he was taking, and he replied that he stopped taking it because he felt so good.

Marie's doctor told her that many bipolar patients quit taking their medication when they start to feel better, but the contrast was so great in her mind between what he looked like in the hospital and what he looked like now she couldn't believe it. Marie could see why he thought he could stop taking it, but she wouldn't do that. She felt stable and better than she had ever felt before; you wouldn't catch her going off her meds. Her problems were solved.

Chapter Thirty-Five

Marie was gone from home for nearly a month. It was so good to be back in her own apartment with her cats. It wasn't possible for her to just lie around and be cured; Marie had to find a job quickly. She naïvely thought that since the new medications made her feel so good her life would straighten up now and everything would be smooth sailing.

Marie felt like she could conquer the world; that she was starting all over again with all the advantages she lacked before. It was painful, but she looked back on all the ambitions she had when she was young; most of them were no longer possible, but Marie hoped it would be possible to start over with a new outlook and new abilities.

She went to the clinic, where the doctor asked her where she had been. "I told you I was going to get some treatment. I went to University and admitted myself to their clinic. They gave me Tegretol, and I am all better."

"So it really works?" He sounded unbelieving.

"Yes, it works, and if you gave it to me years ago I wouldn't have had such a hard time. It would have helped if you had known your medications."

He paused. "I will have to start trying it on some of my patients. I did not realize that it was an option."

"It is, and I am happy to tell you that it has made a real difference in my life."

Now the only problems she had with the clinic were the rude employees and the interminable waits for every aspect of service. But she could get her appointments in the evening, and the drugs were affordable, charged on a sliding scale. She hated going to the clinic, but she counted her blessings and continued to get medication there.

She called Jerri, her friend from school, and said, "Hi, Jerri, it's Marie. I haven't been able to help you with your house for the past few weeks because I've been in the hospital. You see, I have bipolar disorder, and"…Click. Marie thought Jerri would be happy for her when she told her she had found the right medication, finally, and was doing so much better. Evidently not.

Marie felt sad and angry that someone she thought of as a friend could just blow her off like that. It was her first experience with the stigma of the illness and it made her feel helpless to communicate honestly with people. She found that most people did not want to hear about the disorder and didn't want anything to do with her once they found out she had it. She learned to keep her mouth shut.

She had to continue to work as a temporary to pay the bills, but it wasn't steady, and she often felt nervous at the end of the month about making the rent. Finding a new job was hard because she had a hole in her résumé from all the temporary work and from the time spent in the hospital. It didn't look good. When she was downtown, looking for work, she had an idea. Marie went to Caleb's office to catch up with him and to ask a favor.

Caleb was an attorney she often worked with at Child Welfare twenty years before. He was appointed by the court to represent the child in many cases. She also had a year-long affair with him those many years ago. They remained friends she and never lost her deep respect for him. Though they might not see each other often, they always checked in on one another. She was manic at the time of the affair and she hadn't felt guilty about Caleb being married, but now she did.

Caleb was Lincolnesque. He was tall, with a shock of brown hair that fell over his forehead. His smile could be either shy or sly. He knew everyone in town and had a story for each of them. It was annoying to walk down the street with him—you couldn't go two feet before he ran into someone who had to talk with him or he had to talk to.

When she got to his office, she asked, "How have you been?"

He answered, "I still haven't gotten over that loss of my judgeship in family court, but to win I'd have to run as a Republican, and everyone knows I'm a Democrat, so that wouldn't work. How could they expect me to judge fairly if they knew I was lying about my politics? Business is good, though."

"Good. I am sorry you lost the judgeship. I know you are good at it and really look out for the welfare of the children. You know I voted for you. But I understand your feelings about changing parties.

I came here to ask you a favor today. I have this huge hole in my résumé while I was in the hospital and I wondered if you would let me say that I worked here as a paralegal during that time," she said.

"Let me think about that for a minute. I have a better idea. You know Maureen, my partner? I'll want to talk to her about this, but I would like you to come to work here for us, minimum wage, fulltime, until you could find a better job. I know you could help us out, and we could use the help."

"Caleb, that would be a lifesaver for me. I would appreciate it so much. I could count on regular income and not feel like I had to lie to look for another job. But what about your wife? How would she feel about me working here?"

"I make the decisions about who works with me. I'll talk to Maureen this afternoon and call you. I think it would really work out well."

Marie hugged Caleb and left feeling great, but she knew Caleb could be hard to work for. She had met Maureen a couple of times and she seemed like a pleasant, laid-back kind of lady. Even though it didn't pay well, it was the first steady job she had been offered in years, and Marie was really hoping it would work out so she could at least get her résumé in shape, but mostly to have a job to go to every day.

The next day Caleb called, "It's all arranged. Come in Monday morning at 8:30. Maureen thinks it is a great idea. You know B.J., our regular secretary. You will be doing some paralegal work, some correspondence and whatever else Maureen and I come up with. You shouldn't get in her way—you two will get along fine."

"Thank you, Caleb, and thank Maureen for me. I will see you on Monday.

Marie decided since she was so far out from downtown she better purchase a bus card for the month, drive to a park-and-ride, and take the bus into town. That way she wouldn't have to pay parking for her car, which could be pretty pricey. She also wouldn't have to deal with downtown traffic, which was a hassle she could do without.

The first morning it worked out better than she thought it would. The bus driver was having a cup of coffee before he started his run, so when she got on the bus there were a few people already sitting on it, waiting to leave. The driver dashed out to the bus and just assumed that everyone there was a regular. Marie got a free ride downtown and did so every morning she worked. That saved her a dollar a day. After a while, she got so she could fall asleep when she got on the bus, and not wake up until her stop. That gave her an extra forty-five minutes of sleep and made the bus ride painless.

She had to walk about eight blocks from the bus stop to the office, but she wasn't upset about that. Marie had started her diet only a few days before, and the exercise could only help. When she got to the office, she was greeted by B.J., who was a lovely black woman. She didn't seem to resent Marie or feel that she was going to get in B.J.'s way. Somebody had set up a little table for Marie to work at with a typewriter, pens, and a coffee cup. The office was not opulent like so many attorneys' offices; it was more practically furnished. Marie always thought, when she went into one of those offices, that if she were a client, that she was paying for expensive furniture and expensive carpets.

Marie went into Caleb's office to tell him she was there; he greeted her and told her just to help B.J. until he came up with work for her. Maureen was not in yet, and B.J. told her she wouldn't be for quite a while.

She learned the phone etiquette for the office, made copies, and typed a few things for B.J. About 11:30, Maureen came in and greeted her effusively. Maureen was a blonde, extremely attractive woman who also specialized in family law. She talked with Marie and B.J. for a while and then she and Caleb went to lunch.

Marie stayed in for lunch. She was eating around twelve hundred calories a day, so lunch meant something like a can of tuna. She was determined to lose the weight she gained by taking the medications that hadn't done her any good. She wasn't planning to get down to one hundred pounds again—that was too thin, but she thought she would try to diet down to one hundred and thirty pounds. She was upset about her looks and had been buying her "fat clothes" at Goodwill so wasn't happy with her wardrobe. She wanted to be back to a thinner size immediately but she knew it would take time.

After lunch, Caleb sent her to the Courthouse to set some dates for hearings, and then had copying for her to do when she got back. He also asked her to handle some of his correspondence, and was happy with what she did. He said, "You said exactly what I wanted to say, but I couldn't figure out how to say it." Marie was proud of that.

Maureen only had a few things for her to mail. Marie was able to catch the 4:30 bus and get home by 5:30. It was a long day because of the bus rides, but she didn't have to drive in traffic or worry about her car.

It didn't take any time at all for her to discover that Caleb and Maureen had opposite styles. Caleb encouraged his clients to settle out of court, to use arbitrators, to avoid custody fights. Maureen, on the other hand, urged those she worked with to spend as much time as possible in court, and to always contest custody. Marie grew to admire Caleb more, even though he could be tough to work for. One time she used a file to write a letter and then returned it to his desk. All of a sudden, he yelled at her, "Where is the Thompson case?"

Marie said, "It's on your desk."

"No, it isn't. I've looked."

"Yes, it is. I just put it there."

"Look, I didn't hire you to make it difficult. I need that file now!"

Marie went into his office, looked through the files on his desk, pulled out the Thompson file, and handed it to him. "Oh," he said.

This sort of thing happened on a regular basis.

After a couple of months, Maureen got in the habit of saving up all the work she wanted Marie to do until she was ready to leave the office, about 4:30. She would come out of her office, ready to leave, with her arms full of work to be mailed, copied, or typed. "Goodnight, all," she would chirp.

Maureen would sail out of the office, and B.J. would get up to leave, giving Marie a pitying look. “I don’t stay past 4:30.”

Caleb was usually gone by then, so Marie would be left by herself to finish her work.

Chapter Thirty-Six

Marie's relationship with Maureen continued to crater. It seemed to Marie that Maureen didn't care about anyone but herself. Marie got home so late in the evening because of Maureen's schedule that she was shaking from hunger from of her diet and she was ready to eat her own fingers. Once Maureen bustled out of the office, saying to Marie as she left, "I have to leave. It's getting dark outside and my Mercedes is parked in the building next door, so I'll have to be out on the street. It's too dangerous for a woman."

Marie sighed, looking at the pile of work in front of her, and thought of the eight-block walk she had to the bus stop. It would be full dark before she was able to catch her bus.

When Marie made a mistake, Maureen said to her, "Marie, why can't you do anything right?" Marie turned red with embarrassment and anger.

She flounced back to her office, and Marie threw up her hands and headed for the elevator. They were on the ninth floor, and by the time Marie reached the lobby, she knew she really didn't want to walk off the job. It wouldn't be fair to Caleb, and it was no way to build a résumé. So, she squared her shoulders and caught the next elevator up. Marie wondered if she would have turned around if she weren't on her medication.

On Christmas Eve, Caleb wanted to open the office even though every law firm in town was closed. "You never know when a client might need help." B.J. and Marie were a bit disgusted at having to come in on a day they knew wasn't going to be busy, but they couldn't say "No." Maureen wasn't coming in at all.

There was snow on the ground and Marie asked Caleb if she could wear her cowboy boots to keep her feet from freezing at the bus stop. He said, "No, this is still a law office."

So she wore them on the bus and carried nicer shoes into the office. The phone did not ring all day and no one came in. Finally, at two o'clock, Caleb decided to call it a day. He drove B.J. to her car and Marie to her bus stop. They all said "Merry Christmas," and got started on their holiday.

When they returned to the office the day after Christmas, she wrote a memo to Caleb and Maureen, telling them that she was giving notice that she was leaving as soon as she was able to locate another job. Then she set about finding one.

Meanwhile, she finished her diet. She noticed that an antique shop she passed every day on her way to work had a doctor's scale in it. Every morning she stopped and weighed herself on it. Marie never said a word to the proprietor, or him to her, but it was a real help to be able chart her progress. Within three months, she lost to her goal weight, one hundred and thirty pounds. She felt much better about herself and about looking for another job. Now, with a good job, she could buy some new clothes.

In a couple of weeks, she found an ad that sounded promising, so she sent in a résumé that said she had worked for Caleb and Maureen for a year, covering much of the time she was in the hospital and couldn't find work. She gave Caleb as a reference, but not Maureen. Marie got an interview with the law firm that was on the other side of downtown but served by the same bus line.

Caleb told her salacious stories about the founder of the law firm and the Best Little Whorehouse in Texas, but said he would not be involved in the day-to-day. He told her that the firm was in the business of collecting property taxes for the City and that was all he knew.

Marie went to the interview not certain she wanted the job, but when she got there, she was favorably impressed. The offices were not decorated as flamboyantly as most law offices were, and the work of the firm was headed by a woman, Linda. She asked her to be a “team player” so, of course, Marie agreed. The pay was not astronomical, but it beat minimum wage by a good deal. She accepted the position, which would start in two weeks.

Marie felt that her job with Caleb was kind of a “charity” job and was glad to be starting a job that was based on merit. Maureen didn’t seem to mind her leaving; Caleb said he was sorry to see her go, but glad that she had obtained a job that paid more. Marie was glad to be leaving, primarily because of Maureen, but she also felt funny about working for Caleb when she had to take calls for him from his wife, Dora. She knew Dora was a smart woman.

When she reported to her new job, her duties seemed straightforward enough. She was to be an assistant to the man, John, who headed up the collection of delinquent taxes. He had a modest office, and Marie’s desk was right outside. Beyond her desk were eight cubicles, where his people worked for him, making collection calls to people who had not paid their taxes.

What bothered her about the job at first was that according to state law, people over the age of sixty-five could not lose their homes because of tax delinquency. The collectors did not threaten anyone of that age with loss of their homes, but they came as close as they could. They never told them that they were immune from losing their houses. Marie knew that they scared the money out of many older people who really couldn't afford to pay the taxes.

Marie was still smoking at that time, and she took smoke breaks with other employees. It was disconcerting that one employee told her all about his side business that he worked on during hours he was supposed to be working for the law firm. A manager she took breaks with asked her to feel out this employee and find out if he was working on his personal business while he should be working for the law firm. Marie just kept her mouth shut, but she didn't think she should be asked to inform on another employee. She also didn't think the employee should be telling her about his business.

Shortly after she got there, she was working at her desk when the fire alarm sounded. Her job was on the nineteenth floor of a high rise; Marie didn't think, she just grabbed her purse and hustled down nineteen flights of stairs. She stood around in front of the building for about half an hour, then a security guard told her it was just a false alarm. She took the elevator back up to work, and realized that no one else from her job had left. Her boss walked by, and threw out sideways, "You sure wasted a lot of time by leaving." Marie had no intention of being caught in a high-rise fire, but it looked like she had done the wrong thing at that company.

As time went by and Marie settled into her job, her boss, John, started showing his true colors. Marie was his assistant, so she took the brunt of it, though he did to all the women in the firm. He was the worst at sexual harassment she ever encountered. Marie would be standing next to him, talking about something related to the job, when a woman from another division would come in and bend over to get something from the file cabinet.

He would say, "Look at that."

"Doesn't that look good?"

"Wouldn't you like to get ahold of something like that?"

"Mhmmmmm."

Marie and any other women present would simply stand there in silence, not knowing what to say or where to look.

John also had Playboy centerfolds hanging over his desk in his office, and encouraged the other men in the Collections Department to emulate him. Most of them did not, but one also had photos of women in various states of undress hanging on the inside and outside of his cubicle.

All of the women were upset about it, but no one said anything. Marie followed their lead and tried to ignore it, but she found it to be the most degrading situation she had ever been in. His comments were not occasional, but constant, happening several times a day.

Between this and being asked to inform on a fellow employee, Marie really felt that she was in a hostile workplace. But she also knew what it was like not to have a job, so she hung on. She didn't complain to anyone about it, not to Caleb or her family.

Marie kept quiet and just put up with things, but one day John pushed her too far. She couldn't believe she was expected to put up with his behavior. She requested a meeting with the boss, whom she didn't see often, but had been kind to her when she first came to work and had started by catching bronchitis from a fellow employee. Marie hadn't been paid yet and didn't have the money to go to a doctor, but when the boss questioned her about her hacking cough and found out about her situation, loaned her the money to go to the doctor until payday.

At her meeting, Marie said, "I want to tell you how upset it makes me that John talks about sex all day and in front of all the women in his division. We just have to stand there and listen. Couldn't you ask him to stop it?" Marie thought this was a reasonable request to make considering that most of the employees of the firm were women.

Linda stared at her. “I can’t believe that you wasted my time with this stuff. What John talks about is none of your business, and I have never had a complaint about him before. We simply don’t need you here anymore. You are not the team player we asked you to be. Just pack up your stuff and leave.”

Marie was stunned. She did as she was told, packed up her personal belonging and went out to catch the bus. When the bus pulled up, the driver said, “You don’t usually ride this early.”

Marie burst into tears and said, “I just got fired.”

“You get a free ride home, then.”

Chapter Thirty-Seven

When she told people what had happened with her job, they invariably asked her why she didn't sue. Marie didn't think it was a good idea to sue a law firm, and she let it go. The thought of losing two jobs in six months was unbearable.

Marie applied for a temporary position with another firm. As she was being interviewed, the interviewer said she would get the job because her qualifications were excellent. Coincidently, the boss at Marie's last job was the interviewer's next-door neighbor.

The interviewer asked, "What does Linda do there? I've always wondered."

"She runs the place."

"Oh, I didn't know that. I'll let you know about the job tomorrow."

Marie hoped that she wouldn't check up on her references. When the interviewer never called back, her suspicion was Linda had given her a bad review. So it was back to want ads and temp agencies with an updated résumé with a few obvious gaps in her job history. It was beginning to look like it would take a long time to find permanent work. At least this time she was eligible for unemployment compensation.

Marie was to get a nice income tax refund. She waited for her W-2s, and got them all, including Caleb's, but did not receive one from Maureen. When the deadline passed, she called her. Maureen said she was busy, but would get it out soon. Marie waited, and called, and waited some more. At the end of March, she lost patience and called the Internal Revenue Service. Two weeks later the W-2 form was in her mailbox and she filed for her refund.

When she called Caleb and said, “Did you hear what I did? I didn’t get my W-2 from Maureen so I turned her into the IRS and they made her send me one, finally.”

Caleb laughed uproariously. Marie hadn’t realized that Maureen would be fined by the IRS for her dereliction. Caleb said, “It’s about time someone called her out for procrastination.”

Marie continued to attend Mensa events and parties, but she was not attracted to anyone. She wasn’t dating anyone, and that was kind of odd for her. She felt just fine on her own. It had been two years since she gone on a date. Wait, there was one recent date, but it didn’t hardly count. Mark picked her up, took her to a Mensa meeting, drove through a MacDonald’s for some hamburgers, and took her to his place.

When they got there, he asked her to come into the kitchen with him. He said, “I always eat over the sink because that way I don’t get any dishes or the table dirty.”

She looked at him quizzically, but he really meant it. So they ate their food standing over the sink. It was one of the more unromantic dates she had ever been on, and she made it clear that there wouldn’t be a second. That was weird, she thought. Maybe I don’t need to date. It was times like these she missed Jackie the most, because she didn’t have a friend she could call up and who would be incredulous about such a thing and then laugh with her about it.

She spent several months looking for work, living on both unemployment and working temporary, because unemployment lasted longer if supplemented with work. She was getting discouraged when she saw an ad that she had seen several times before, asking for someone who had an education in the social sciences, or was a paralegal.

The name of the company was Political Research, and they wanted a background in teaching or writing. The job sounded perfect to her, but she noticed that she had seen the ad run about every six months. She knew there had to be something wrong if there was such a large turnover.

Marie decided to try it, anyway, and see what the situation was. She sent in her résumé and got an appointment. By this time, she had moved right into their neighborhood. Although it was kind of scary when she got an interview, Marie put on her navy blue suit and drove there, surprised at how small the place was. The picture in the phone book made it look enormous. It actually looked like a tiny little White House.

Warily, Marie went in, and the receptionist seated her in the foyer while she got the president of the company to talk with her. Waiting, she couldn't help but notice that the place was unnaturally quiet for workplace where people turned out books: she couldn't hear a sound.

Surprisingly the president was a fifty-year old woman named Judy. Judy explained that the company put out yearbooks with the members of Congress and state legislatures mainly for libraries, educational institutions, and lobbying groups, and anyone else who might want to have information about lawmakers. They also had a service, and this is where Marie would come in.

Any subscriber to the books and the company's monthly newsletter could call in and ask about any government function and get an answer. Many people subscribed to this service. It sounded like an interesting job, too. Marie didn't ask any questions or get any answers about the turnover, but she was grateful to get the job, which would start the next Monday. One thing that sounded strange was the requirement that she wear blue every day.

Marie made a quick trip to the thrift shop over the weekend and got blue blazers and jackets, and a couple of blue skirts. She thought she could manage with the rest of her wardrobe.

On Monday, she showed up, curious as to what she would learn. The publisher, a man in his eighties who had founded the company, introduced her to the editors and writers who made up the staff. The other woman she would work with was a young woman just out of college and paralegal school named Camilla.

Camilla was short and slender, with long dark hair and dark eyes. Attractive, but didn't try to get by on that. She caught on quickly and worked hard. In no time, Marie could tell they would be a good team.

All they had to work with was a directory of phone numbers for all Federal agencies and a few reference works, most of them brought in by Camilla or Marie. It was obvious they had hired them because they were conversant with how the government worked and knew where to go for answers to our client's questions. They handled dozens of inquiries a day; it was fast-paced and fun.

From listening to employees already on the job and from personal observation, it became obvious that Judy was operating with a bad case of paranoid personality disorder. She was convinced that the workers in the company were out to destroy it, even though that made no sense. She sneaked around trying to hear conversations, and interpreted what she heard or saw as being negative for the workplace.

The other employees told them that the turnover rate was one hundred percent per year, that people were fired for no reason constantly, and no amount of good work and reliability would guarantee your job. The publisher, however, was almost senile, and all decisions about how the company was run by

Judy, who was in a long-standing affair with him. All of this seemed unlikely, but Marie and Camilla could see the atmosphere in which they worked, and two weeks after they were hired, one of the writers offended in some way and was fired.

Realizing that she needed a writer, Judy held a meeting and asked which of the staff members had knowledge and an interest in the Supreme Court. Marie raised her hand, and Judy told her she would be writing the Court column in the monthly newsletter from then on. This meant that Marie would pick an interesting case, summarize it, and explain its meaning in a one-page article. There would be no extra pay and she would have to do the work at home, because there wasn't time during regular hours.

It didn't seem like a good deal, but Marie was fascinated by the Court, and she knew it would give her writing experience. She always wanted to be a writer, but she was never before given a chance. When she graduated from college, there were no job openings for women writers, so she hadn't really thought about preparing to be a writer.

She did the work carefully, and the peak of her experience came when she realized in the case she was summarizing the clerk had used the work "desegregation" when he meant "segregation." When she finalized her article, she indicated that it was a mistake. The head writer said, "You can't just show that this is a mistake, you have to verify it with the Court."

"Paul, anyone reading this sentence can see it is a mistake."

"I don't care, we have to be accurate. Call the Court."

Marie felt a little silly calling the Court, but the secretary at the Court was pleasant; she checked with the clerk and got back to her right away. She said, "Yes, of course that was a mistake, he certainly didn't mean to say "desegregation" there. When we reprint the case, we will correct it. But I want you to know that no one else caught that, not even the New York Times guy."

Judy wasn't impressed, but Marie was. She had to pat herself on the back.

One morning Camilla came into the office with a funny look on her face. "Marie, what were you just talking about?"

"I was raving about the latest Supreme Court decision. I think it was a bad decision and I was just expressing that opinion."

"When I walked past the boss' office Judy was telling him that you were complaining about what a terrible place this was to work and how you couldn't wait to leave."

"Camilla, you know I wouldn't be saying that. I guess it doesn't matter, though, what you say."

After about a year and a half, Camilla and Marie had become quite a team. They made the clients happy with the efficient, accurate answers they gave them. It was a surprise, then, when Camilla was called into Judy's office at 4:50 on a Friday night. That is how people were routinely fired. Judy and the publisher would call them in to the president's office and talk for twenty minutes about why the person was being fired. By the time, they were finished everyone would have left for the day. Marie thought the idea was that by Monday everyone should have forgotten about him or her.

When she got home that night, she waited for Camilla's call. Camilla did call her and it was obvious she had been crying; it was also obvious she was crying because of anger. Marie asked, "What did they tell you?"

"They said I wasn't being cooperative enough. I asked for example of me not being cooperative and they didn't give me any—they just said I wasn't working out."

Marie was angry, too, that they would fire her when she had only done top-notch work for them. She couldn't understand what good it would do them to let her go. "Camilla, it's good they fired you. You are young and have good degrees. You will be able to get a job in no time. I am going to miss you, though. I wonder who I will have to train now."

"You are still stuck there. I won't be looking for a job right away—I hadn't told you this yet, but Clark and I are planning on being married. I'm just going to take off and plan the wedding now."

"That's great!" Marie exclaimed. "Let me know how it goes, and be sure to invite me."

"I will!"

Chapter Thirty-Eight

Judy didn't hire anyone to take Camilla's place; she just moved a writer over to help Marie out. So Marie didn't have to do much training with him, mostly just bailing him out when he was stuck.

At Mensa, Marie met Stewart, famous throughout the national organization of Mensa for his satirical writings in group newsletters. Absolutely nothing escaped his pen, and his writings were quite controversial. People either loved them or hated them. Marie had been reading his comedy for years and thought he was pure funny.

He was a member of her local Mensa chapter, but she had not met him before. When he came to a function one Saturday night, they hit it off immediately. They talked about his writing, and she asked him, "What are you doing now?"

He said, "I'm just doing freelance writing. I used to work for the newspaper but they let me go."

Since she was so attracted to him, Marie asked, "Are you married?"

"I'm separated right now, getting a divorce. I'm living with my sister."

As they talked, he put his arms around her and pulled her to him. She stood in front of him, and they discussed politics, finding out that they were on the same page with that. They had the same sense of humor.

They both liked to walk, and made a date to meet the next day in the park Marie went every day. This evolved into a daily activity, and as they walked and talked, before they knew it they were an item. Marie ghost-wrote a couple of stories with him, and he encouraged her to write more on her own.

Marie started writing stories for the local newsletter. Some were picked up by other newsletters and within a few months, her writing was in demand from Boston to Albuquerque.

Her stories were about her family, such as her grandmother who had homesteaded on the Oklahoma prairie or her other grandmother who survived the monstrous Galveston hurricane. Without Stewart's encouragement, Marie didn't think she would have ever tried to get published.

The relationship did not always run smoothly. Stewart needed her to motivate him to look for a job, to get new glasses, or even go to the doctor. Marie got tired of having to tell an adult what to do and then having to drive him wherever he needed to go. He wouldn't do anything unless she went with him.

If they had a disagreement about anything, Stewart would refuse to talk about it and would storm out, throwing things as he went, and telling her, "I never want to see you again."

Of course, the next day he would show up, perfectly happy, and ready to go on. Because of this, they never talked about any issues they had. For example, he often made sexually explicit remarks to Marie about women he saw on the street or in the grocery store. Marie found this insulting, and calmly asked him to stop.

"I don't see why I should. I'm not hurting anyone; I'm just expressing my opinion."

Then he stormed out. Marie didn't know how to fix that, though she tried to talk to him calmly, he always got upset and left.

At work, nothing changed. A writer was fired because her son broke his neck in a motorcycle accident and she had to take off work to care for him. This made all the employees angry, but they couldn't do anything about it. Stewart and Marie came up with a prank they couldn't resist.

Since the publisher gave Judy a new Cadillac every year, she had simply parked her old car in the parking lot of the business about ten years before, and it just sat there, on four flat tires, slowly disintegrating. Noticing the bright red stickers her apartment manager affixed to cars that were not being maintained, threatening to tow them, Marie asked her if she could have one to play a joke on someone. The manager grinned and gave her one.

At three o'clock, the next morning Marie and Stewart went to the company and placed it on Judy's old car. Of course, Judy was parked in a private parking lot and no one could tell her to move it.

The next day at work Marie passed the word about what she had done the night before. Everyone watched to see what would happen, if anything. To the employees' great surprise, late in the morning a tow truck showed up and towed Judy's car. She moved it because she thought she had to. They kept straight faces, but it was the one of the only times they actually pulled something off.

Later on, when the head writer was fired, he came back in the middle of the night and used a baseball bat to demolish the eagles that sat atop the pillars that surrounded the building. The owner was so prepared and accustomed to that form of vengeance he had them replaced by noon.

Toward the end of the year, it was time for the company to put out an international yearbook containing statistics on every country in the world, plus a description of each one. This was too much for the regular writers, so contract writers were hired.

Marie went to the new manager in charge, "Jeff, I have a boyfriend who is an accomplished writer, but I know we can't tell the bosses we are in a relationship, because they won't hire him then."

"Just bring in a writing sample and I won't tell them anything about who he is."

Stewart was hired right away but it was embarrassing to Marie that he had trouble making his deadlines. She told Jeff, "Give him deadlines that are two weeks prior to when the article is needed." It gave Marie insight as to why Stewart had lost his regular job with the newspaper.

By this time, it was getting close to the end of the year. Each Christmas, Judy fired someone just because she could. Marie waited until two weeks before Christmas to buy presents for her family, not knowing if she would make it through the season. However, the Friday before Christmas, at 4:50 in the afternoon, Judy called her into her office.

Marie knew what that meant, and she was angry. She had worked there for two and a half years, had done a great job despite their criticism and now was going to be fired for some obscure reason.

She went into the office and sat down.

Judy started off, "Marie, you have been here for a while, but things are just not working out with you."

Marie interrupted," Are you firing me?"

"Yes, unfortunately, we are."

Marie refused to sit there and listen to the convoluted reasons as to why she was being fired. She stood up and left the room, and started packing up her desk. She was angry, and made a lot of noise and commotion. No one in the building missed what she was doing. Everyone was still there, working, so they didn't get to let her go in secret. Marie left with the others, and outside they said "good-bye." Several of them told her "not to worry about it, it wasn't her fault."

Marie was angry and disgusted, but got over it quickly when she realized it was just her turn to be fired. She couldn't have done anything to prevent it, and she didn't do anything to cause it. It was just time to put on her job-looking shoes again.

When Stewart called in for his writing assignments the next Monday, the amount of work had been doubled. Nothing was ever said to them, but it was just understood that Marie was being given contract work under the table by Jeff. She did the work for months and she and Stewart split the checks. She found it hilarious that she was still working for the company, still being paid by them, and the bosses didn't know it.

This time Marie wanted to find a writing job. She had her Supreme Court column as writing samples, and she had also written several shorter articles about various subjects for the company newsletter. Now she also had the international articles. A writing position was what she hoped for, but was not limiting herself to one.

After Stewart and she finished the contract writing, she went on unemployment and he also needed a job. While looking for herself, Marie found an ad for a writer to write a corporate history for a well-known company. "Stewart, this is something that you could do, and the job would last for months.'

"I sure could, and I could use the money, too. What do they want?"

"Writing samples and a résumé."

Marie and Stewart got them together and mailed them off to the address in the ad. It wasn't two days before they got a response on Marie's answering machine, now that she was able to afford one. It made her life easier, especially when she was looking for work. They asked Stewart to come in for an interview.

"I don't know where the place is where he wants me to interview." Stewart said.

"I have a map."

"Oh, I'm no good with maps. Will you drive me there?"

"I think you can get there by yourself."

"Please, Marie, I don't want to be late and I have a terrible time finding places."

"Okay, Stewart, but I always have to go to my job interviews by myself."

On the appointed day, Marie drove Stewart to the interview, and then sat outside in the car for an hour. When Stewart came out, he was ecstatic. "I got the job."

"That's great. Does it pay well?'

"Yes, it does, and it will last about a year. The headquarters of the company are in Waco, so there's some travel involved."

"I'm so glad you got the job."

"I hope you find one soon."

This episode had convinced her that she could no longer support Stewart—it was like having a two-year old around, and she didn't want a child or to have to tell someone what to do all the time, so Marie told him good-bye. He didn't believe her at first and kept showing up, but she finally convinced him of her decision. She wasn't surprised when he told her a year later that he missed a bonus by being six weeks late on the deadline.

Chapter Thirty-Nine

Marie's unemployment checks were close to running out when she saw the ad for a writer. She had never heard of the company, but it was only a mile or so from her apartment. Her first thought was, this would be too good to be true. That didn't stop her from applying, though.

Marie sent off the copy of her résumé that emphasized her writing experience along with the writing samples they requested. Within a few days, she got a call from Ruth, the person who would be her supervisor if hired, asking her to come in for an interview.

Marie was stoked. This sounded like her dream job and it didn't include riding the bus or driving a long distance. However, she didn't get too carried away—her last job sounded perfect for her and look at how that had turned out. She went to the interview both excited and skeptical.

At the company, she happily noticed that it was not unnaturally silent. In fact, there was quite a bit of noise in the building. She sat in the lobby shaking with nerves, juggling her purse, her coffee, and a folder with transcripts and other papers. When Ruth came out to shake her hand, it was the coffee she dropped. They both laughed, but Marie wanted to cry.

She followed Ruth into the office. After they were seated, Ruth said, "This job mainly consists of writing and editing material, called syllabi, which accompany continuing education videos made by healthcare professionals. I see that you taught and wrote and your paralegal experience would come into play here, too. Do you think this is something you would be interested in doing?"

"This sounds like a perfect job and I am happy to show you my transcripts."

Ruth showed her samples of the work they did, and explained there were two deadlines a month they had to meet. Sometimes the person doing the video supplied them with information, which they edited, and sometimes they were on their own to write something to accompany the video. They covered all subjects from radiology to long-term care.

To Marie, the job sounded fascinating. There were drawbacks that she could see right away—the work was done in a large room that accommodated about fifty other people, so naturally the noise level was high. They had two bosses; a registered nurse and the head of the producers, and they had to make both of them happy. And then there were the two deadlines a month. She could see it was a challenge, but she really hoped she would get the job, and told Ruth so.

"There's only one thing, though, I have to ask you not to call Judy at Political Research for a reference, but you can call the others I have listed."

Marie held her breath.

"You worked there for two and a half years, so you couldn't have been that bad. I'll just skip her when I check your references. I see you have given me three others."

Marie breathed again, in relief.

It was only two days later that Marie got the call she was waiting for—Ruth calling to tell her she got the job. Marie showed up a couple of days later, ready to start a new job, but a little apprehensive, too. Ruth was her supervisor, and Caroline was her boss. Shari was the program director and all of them seemed nice. Joy was the nurse. At least Marie didn't have to look around to see who was listening before she said anything.

There were some bumps in the road. Marie had little experience with computers, and had never used a mouse. However, in a couple of weeks she would be formatting articles with a desktop publishing program. It didn't sound possible to Marie, but Ruth assured her that she would learn that fast.

After a couple of weeks, she was on her computer doing amazing things when the pain of a kidney stone hit her. The doctor told her that she had to wait a week to remove the stone because of insurance rules and that it wouldn't be possible for her to work while she waited. She was embarrassed to miss work right after being hired.

She asked Ruth, "Can you bring some work by my apartment so I can do it at home?"

Ruth said, "I'll check with Shari and see what we should do."

Shari called her at home. "Don't worry; we'll pay you while you are off. A kidney stone is not something you can plan." Marie did as much work as she could for Ruth, but it was a big weight off her mind to know that she would be paid while she was sick.

After a week, she had surgery to remove the stone, and was back at work in a few days. She made up for some of the time missed by working cxtra hours, but no one ever asked her to. Marie became adept at the program used to format the articles they published, and also learned the style of writing they expected her to use. She was pulling her weight within two months. There was still a lot to learn, but at least the bosses were happy with her.

Nothing about her job resembled working at Political Research and Marie found herself happy at work and at home. She wasn't dating anyone at the time, and she didn't feel like she needed to be. Concentrating on her work was keeping her busy.

She found out what it was like working for a good company. The dress code consisted of only looking as good as you needed to if someone were coming from the outside to work with you, keeping in mind that in such a large room someone always had a visitor coming. Your hours were what you needed to work to get your work done; you started and stopped when you needed to. There were no requirement to wear a certain color and you could wear pants.

The company supplied hot lunches, prepared by a chef, at cost for the employees, so there was no need to go out for lunch; that saved time and effort and meant employees got good food, not fast food. Marie and Ruth generally worked about fifty hours a week getting their packets of syllabi out; it didn't worry them that it was more than forty hours. The place was so pleasant to work in that Marie was fine with working extra hours. Also, there were those two deadlines they had to meet. Marie was aghast when she learned that missing a deadline would cost the company thirty thousand dollars in extra postage to get the syllabi to the customers by airdate. That was a motivator.

There was a fly in the ointment, of course. Ruth had some down days—some of them so bad Caroline had to send her home. She would cry uncontrollably at her desk and tell her troubles to anyone, whether they wanted to listen or not. Sometimes she would go out onto the front steps and sit and cry. Once the nurse found her, sobbing, crouched under the sink in the ladies' room.

Caroline asked Marie, "Are you ready to take over if Ruth leaves now?"

Marie, shocked, said, "No, I don't know enough about the detail of the preparation of the packets to go to the printers yet."

Marie had once had a friend, Anita, who fell into a deep depression. Her job counseled her, sponsored her stay at a hospital, and paid for her therapy and drugs. That gave Marie an idea.

"Ruth works hard and does a really good job. Instead of firing her, why not tell her that you will fire her unless she gets some treatment?"

Caroline said, "That's a good idea. I'll talk to Shari about it."

Marie was relieved; she really wasn't ready to take over the job, and she didn't want to see Ruth fired over what seemed to be depression. Slowly, over the next few months, Ruth had fewer and fewer meltdowns and seemed happier at work, so it seemed to be working.

After a few months, Caroline came over to Marie's desk and asked, "Why didn't you tell me that the syllabi were late this month?"

"What! I didn't know anything about it. You'll have to ask Ruth."

When Ruth came in later in the day, Marie told her what Caroline said.

"They weren't late. I turned them in on time."

Ruth went to Caroline's desk and was told, "the syllabi went out late and when the printers were asked why the extra postage was needed, they said it was because the writers turned them in late."

After much checking, it turned out that the printers got behind in their work because their boss was sick. Marie was glad she wasn't in charge when she saw how many people were unhappy over this.

Marie's spirits had improved over having a job that she truly enjoyed and found a challenge, but didn't feel that the bosses were trying to sabotage here as she had in her last job.

She continued to go to her Mensa activities and to enjoy having friends both at work and on the weekends. She also took the time to go to Camilla's wedding that June.

Chapter Forty

Marie worked at MedPrime for a year when the crazy man hit the Federal Building. That day started out as a normal workday, with Marie editing her latest project. Ruth was not in yet because she liked to come in late and stay late, and the producers were all working on their various programs. Many people were in the room, and each of the producers had his or her own television to help monitor shows. The office buzzed with activity, until people around her gasped and a wave of commotion stirred through the room. The producer a couple of desks over angled her TV so Marie could see. The whole front half of a building was gone, open to the elements. The newsman was explaining it was the Federal Building in downtown Oklahoma City.

People on TV were running, others sitting on the curbs, many of them bleeding. The scene was chaos, almost impossible to take in. No one knew why the building exploded, who was injured, or who was killed. Work stopped in the room except for the immediate, got-to-get-this-done-today work.

Everyone gathered around televisions and to watch the slow progress of extricating survivors from the building, by ladder or fire truck and also the recovery of the bodies. After about an hour, Marie saw ambulances from Norman helping and for the first time realized how big it all was.

Marie didn't have any friends or relatives working there, but didn't know if someone she knew might have been there to conduct business. It would take hours to find out if anyone of the company's employees' loved ones were missing or dead. Everyone waited in dread.

It upset Marie when the news people told kids home from school that if their parent or parents didn't come home from work, they should call a relative or friend, or, if they didn't have anyone to call, they could use a number they gave them to call. Marie imagined herself and her brother and sisters sitting at home, waiting for someone to come home when they were children.

Marie was able to concentrate for a while and got some work done, but not a lot. She heard Connie Chung ask, "Is Oklahoma City able to handle such a terrible tragedy?"

That made her angry, since the City had to guard against F-5 tornadoes and was probably one of the best-prepared cities in the country for a crisis. That was a put-down she would never forget.

About four in the afternoon, Craig, one of the technical guys, came in to talk to his boss.

"I heard from my mom's co-workers. Everyone in her department is safe, but she went to the credit union about the time the bomb went off and no one has seen her since. I need to go to the site and see what is going on."

"Take as much time as you need. I hope you find her all right," Shari, the program director, said.

After that, they all drifted home except for a few who had work to finish. Marie made it a point to drive past her childhood home, which was less than a mile from downtown, and saw broken and cracked windows all up and down the block, and in the home she grew up in. It made her sad and brought home the force of the bomb.

It was hard to get any work done as the days went by. They kept up with conditions by keeping the televisions on all day, and snatching time to work. Everyone, including the citizens of the City, was exhausted. In the evenings and at night they watched television until midnight, and then got up early to catch up on the news before work. Marie heard a tired newsman say.

"The dogs are discouraged, because all the survivors they have found have been dead." She laughed, but knew he was so exhausted he didn't even realize what he said.

Craig's mother wasn't found until the twelfth day, her body buried under a huge pile of debris. Craig was paid the whole time he was off, and they didn't deduct any sick or vacation time. The morning of the funeral, Shari had breakfast catered to his family.

Slowly they weaned themselves from the televisions and got back into a routine. All of them knew they had to go on. But there was no one in the City who didn't know someone who had been touched by senseless event. And it was all random. It made no sense.

After all the weird places Marie worked, it made her happy to work in a place that valued its employees and treated them so well. It inspired her to work as many hours as necessary and to make the product as high quality as possible.

Marie hadn't been spending much time with her parents, because it seemed that she clashed with her father whenever she tried to interact with them. It made her sad that she couldn't see her mother more often, but she talked to her often on the phone. Then, one day, it hit her that her mother hadn't called her in a while—she had done all the calling.

She called her mother and set an evening for her to visit. When she got there, everything looked normal except that her mother seemed subdued. Marie and she talked for a while, and her mother seemed vague, not really there. The only thing animating her was her favorite TV show, *Lawrence Welk*. "I watch him every night. I can't wait for him to come on."

Marie said, "Haven't you already pretty much seen all his shows?"

"I don't think so. I can't remember them if I have." Finally, Marie asked, "What book are you reading?"

All her life, her mother had bemoaned the fact that she didn't get to read enough because she was so busy with childcare and housework. Almost every night, though, she had managed to sneak in a chapter of a book.

Her mother looked confused.

"I don't know why, but I haven't read anything in a long time. It's funny, because I used to like it so much. Now I just don't seem interested."

After her visit, Marie called her sister, Shirley, who got along with their father because she was careful not to disagree with him. She asked, "What is going on with the parents? It doesn't seem right at all with Mother."

"I have been putting off notifying all of you until I was sure. I have an appointment with Mother and her doctor. I think she has Alzheimer's disease."

"Oh no. Maybe she is just tired or depressed. I can't believe that."

"Well, you remember how it was with her mother."

"Yes, I do. And that's why I don't want to believe that it is true. I know she isn't acting right. Thanks for taking this on, and please keep me updated."

Marie was devastated at the thought of her mother having Alzheimer's disease. They all remembered how their mother tried so hard to care for her mother when she had the illness. Her father had retired by this time and wanted to travel all the time and take her away, so she was unable to see her mother for days. Susie told her children she felt bad every day that she had to miss seeing and caring for her mother.

Her grandmother had lost all connection with her children and reverted to childhood. She became helpless, finally spending her time with a baby doll. Then she was diagnosed with breast cancer. Marie remembered her mother calling and saying, “Marie, I just don’t know how long I can take this. Mother is suffering and it just gets worse and worse.”

“I am so sorry you have to go through all this,” Marie sympathized.

The children wished they could help, but they knew there was nothing anyone could do.

In 1976, there was a swine flu epidemic, and an effort to inoculate everyone in the country. It was determined afterwards the shots were fatal to some frail, elderly patients. Marie’s grandmother was one of them—she died the evening of the day she received her shot.

Marie’s mother called each of them, “Marie, your grandmother died yesterday evening. I want you to know that it is mostly a relief to me, because I knew it had to happen soon and it is finally over for her. I am certainly not going to sue the government over that vaccine. I’ll let you know when the funeral is.”

Later, when they all gathered for the funeral, Susie said to her, “I am glad that she died, there was nothing more for her, but losing your mother leaves a real hole in your life. There will never be another person who loves you in the same way as she did.”

Marie remembered those words as she thought about the future and waited to hear about the appointment.

Chapter Forty-One

Shirley called the next day. "The doctor confirmed it. Mother has Alzheimer's disease. Daddy is furious with me for getting the diagnosis. Even though he lives with her and has watched her decline, he refuses to believe it. Her mother had it, but he won't acknowledge she has it. I have been spending more time with them than you have. I've seen that she has almost stopped cooking and cleaning. Daddy does all the housework that gets done now. That usually means they eat frozen dinner. I will let Ann, Tim, and Nancy know and then we can talk about it."

"What can we do? We can't let them live like that but if he won't admit it…"

"I'll call Meals on Wheels and see if they will bring lunches to them. That will at least give them one decent meal a day."

Marie had to admit it to herself now, and she knew it was going to be difficult. Her father had spent most of his life in denial of life's realities, and being sheltered from them by his wife. Getting him to find help for Mother was going to be hard.

Shirley called her back in a couple of days. "I am so frustrated. I called Meals on Wheels and they went out there. Daddy wouldn't open the storm door and cursed them out. He said he would never let them in, he didn't need them, and didn't want them around."

"I was afraid of that."

"I guess all we can do is stay in touch with Mother's doctor and try to monitor the situation," Marie said.

"I am not comfortable with that," said Shirley. "She needs help and we need to get it for her."

"I don't know what we are going to do."

Shirley called a service that helps the elderly with cleaning and cooking, and again, Daddy wouldn't let them in and cursed them for coming. From then on, Tim, Shirley, Marie, and especially Nancy, visited in turn and tried to make sure things were going well. On occasion, their mother would call one of them, but would say, for example, "I have taken a job working for a man, but I don't know his name."

Each time they visited, their mother drifted further and further from them and she lost more and more weight. They were all concerned for her, but could not convince their father to do anything.

Finally, one weekend Marie got a frantic call from Shirley. Their father called her and said,

"The Edmond Police told me that I have to put Mother in a home immediately."

Marie responded, "The police! What do they have to do with it?

"It seems that Mother has been 'going for walks' for several weeks and getting lost. Daddy has been calling the police and they have been going out in force, even using helicopters, to find her. Last week she disappeared in a thunderstorm, barefoot, and it took them hours to find her. The cops told him he was mistreating her and they would not put up with it any longer."

"Oh my god. He never told us about this. So now we have to find a place for her right away?"

"Yes, by next week. I've called everyone and they will be here by tomorrow night. Meanwhile, I'll get Daddy started with Medicaid and ask about places for Mother."

By the next night, all the siblings from Texas and Oklahoma gathered at the family home. Shirley found out that Medicaid would pay for their mother's care in a nursing home, and there was only one place in the area that took people with Alzheimer's disease and had any vacancies. It was all the way across Oklahoma City, but it was the best they could do. The next day they made arrangements to tour the nursing home.

The home was awful. The walls were institutional beige and the floors were brown tile. Each room housed two people who a shared bathroom. Each patient had a closet and dresser of her own. It was clean and well maintained, but the inmates wandered around like lost souls in hell.

They either didn't speak, or they babbled. Their clothes were mismatched, and they shuffled like the damned. Their hair was uncombed and some of the women had tried to apply makeup, making them look like clowns. The kids were horrified by the place.

Outside, they shared their misgivings, but since they had watched having experienced similar problems with their grandmother, they knew this was their mother's future. They also knew this was the only place that could take her. It made them all sad, but they knew they didn't have a choice. Shirley and their father filled out the necessary papers, including a no-resuscitate form. Their father was reluctant to sign this, but the nursing home insisted that he do so. With no choice, he signed.

The next day the family took her there and left her. She continuously begged, "I want to go home."

She had been saying that for weeks, so they weren't sure what home was to her. Did she mean the home she raised her children in? Or her childhood home in Houston? It was heartbreaking to leave her in a place like that, but as Shirley said, “At least we know she can’t escape and get lost again.” That was the only thing that comforted them.

From that day on, Peter got up every morning, put on his suit, and drove across town to the home. He sat beside his wife, who he expected to be dressed in a nice dress and high heels. The staff fixed her up every morning. For a while, she could converse with him, but after a few weeks, her language degenerated into babble.

The first time Marie visited her; her mother looked at her questioningly and asked,

“Aren’t you my sister?”

“No,” Marie answered, “I’m your daughter.”

“Then I don’t know you,” she said. Marie was the only one of the girls who looked like her mother’s side of the family.

Susie had to miss all of the activities scheduled for the residents because her husband visited with her daily and sat with her all day. He refused to miss a day or let her engage in activities without him. “If I didn’t come every day or let her join the activities, that would be leaving her alone and I can’t do that.”

Marie and the others tried to explain to him that it would probably be easier for him if he would find some activities outside of the facility and let her enjoy the ones the home planned for her. He couldn’t grasp it.

Marie visited her often, but it seemed pointless. Her mother didn’t know who she was, couldn’t converse, and was lost in her own world. While she was in the nursing home, the first drug for Alzheimer’s disease came out. In consultation with the doctor, Suzie’s children decided not to put her on it. While it might snap her back into sanity for a while, she would inevitability fade back to the condition she was in now, and they would have to go through the same process again.

~*~

Gazing at her desk calendar at work one day, Marie realized that it had been twenty-five years since she started smoking. She was unhappy with the habit for years, but completely unable to quit cold turkey. She tried many times, but always ended up going to the Seven-Eleven at three in the morning to buy cigarettes.

Now nicotine gum could be sold without a prescription and Marie decided to try again. She chewed the gum like a maniac and sucked on Fireballs, a hot cinnamon candy. To her delight, though it was the hardest thing she had ever did, within a month she had quit.

Caroline, her boss, was incredulous and stated, "If you can quit smoking, I guess I can. I didn't believe that I could before I saw you do it. Now I have to."

It was hard, but Marie continued to stay away from cigarettes from then on. She would not have believed that within five years she would not remember how strong her cravings were. She was happy to be free of her addiction and wished she could have kicked it sooner. Of course, she became addicted to the gum, but she was free of cigarettes.

Chapter Forty-Two

At MedPrime the workload expanded so Ruth and Marie got permission to hire a third person. They hired Charlotte, but she didn't seem to enjoy the job. She wanted to write, but didn't want to do the less-enjoyable parts of the job such as filing and proofing, which irritated Marie. But it was a big help to have assistance with the writing.

At the nursing home, their mother continued to lose cognition and physical abilities, becoming clumsy, mute, incontinent, and having difficulty swallowing. Marie and the others knew when she lost the ability to swallow they would have a tremendous fight with their father, because he would want a stomach tube for feeding inserted to keep her alive, but she had told them many times, "If I am ever in that shape, I don't want that kind of care. Just let me go."

They wanted to be true to her wishes, and they knew that an Alzheimer's patient could live years with a stomach tube, completely helpless and unknowing. She always said that was her nightmare.

The manager of the nursing home called Marie. She said, "You know we have been letting your father eat lunch here with your mother, for free, because we didn't think he was eating properly, and she was getting distracted and forgetting to eat. We thought this might help her to eat."

Marie said, "That is so kind of you. I'm sure it helps mother and we really appreciate it."

The manager answered, "It worked well for a short time, but he got irritated with the manners of the other patients, and became so angry he threw food at them. We can't allow that kind of behavior around our patients, so he was told he couldn't eat with his wife anymore.

"I know you all can't do anything about his behavior, and we don't expect you to, but he does lose control at times. I have to tell you that he slapped a nurse's aide last week, and we cannot tolerate that. I told him he would have to leave and not come back if he did that again," the manager said.

"Oh my god," Marie said, "is she going to sue?"

"No, she was pretty upset, but she understands the condition your father is in."

"What a relief," Marie said.

The children felt they had to do everything to keep their mother in the nursing home where she would be safe, but their father was sabotaging that. If the manager banned him from the nursing home, he would likely take her home and try to care for her there, which would be impossible. They were grateful that the manager was understanding and stayed in touch with her in case she had complaints. All they could really do was to apologize.

For Christmas, their father wanted to do something special. He asked Nancy to host Christmas dinner for all of the family in El Reno. Everyone would converge on the small town, eat dinner and open presents, and then stay in a motel before we returned to our homes the next day. He checked mother out of the nursing home and drove her to El Reno.

When mother got there, all of her children and grandchildren were waiting for her. She seemed confused and withdrawn, eyes dull and vacant, showing no sign that she recognized anyone. She didn't know it was Christmas; and was oblivious to what was going on around her. When the family sat down to dinner, it got quieter and she seemed calmer.

All of a sudden Daddy yelled, “Goddamnit, somebody help her!” Everyone at the table who had been quietly talking before, jumped and looked around, startled. What was wrong? Finally, Tim, who was sitting next to mother, realized that she had picked up her sweet potatoes with her hand to eat them. He switched places with Nancy so she could feed their mother. The atmosphere became somber after the outburst.

The family never tried anything like that again. About the time the manager of the nursing home told the children it was becoming almost impossible for their mother to eat, she suffered a massive stroke and died. Marie felt just as her mother did when her grandmother died. She would always miss her mother, but she was not sad she had died.

The next Thanksgiving and Christmas, all the family gathered at their father’s house for dinner. Their father was still grieving, but he said nothing about his wife or about missing her. Marie thought it was nice to see Tim and Nancy again so soon.

A week after Christmas, Marie got a phone call from their father’s doctor. “Your father has to be out of his house in three weeks and the family isn’t helping him at all. Where do you expect him to go?”

“What?”

“You mean you don’t know that Peter has sold his house and has to be out in three weeks?

“I haven’t heard anything like that.” Marie said.

Marie went to her father’s house and got him to tell her about it. He verified what the doctor said, that he had sold the house and needed to find another place to live and move within three weeks.

“Why didn’t you tell us?”

“I didn’t think you would be interested.”

“Where are you planning to move?”

“I don’t know, maybe Tim will let me live with him in San Antonio.”

“Don’t you think you should have asked? Never mind,” Marie said, “I’ll call everyone and we’ll figure it out.”

Shirley got a call from Marie, telling her about the situation. Tim, Shirley, Nancy and her got together and started sorting their parents’ belongings that weekend. Tim told his father that he couldn’t take him in because he and Lowell were looking for new jobs and they didn’t know where they would end up. Tim told his sisters there was no way he could tolerate having their father living with them.

Marie knew she couldn’t take him in, and neither would Shirley. During the next week, Nancy found a pleasant assisted living home that he could afford in El Reno.

“Well,” Tim said, “We probably can’t do any better than that. Nancy can keep an eye on him and it is good of her to volunteer. I can’t do it, and I know Marie can’t.

Shirley spoke up, “I don’t have the patience either.”

They presented it to their father as a *fait accompli* and at a frantic pace, because they had to work at their jobs during the week, then spend the weekend traveling to his home and packing his things and moving him. He wouldn’t hear of using a moving company and Tim had to drive up from San Antonio three weekends in a row.

It fell to Nancy to get him settled in. She reported that he was refusing to socialize, to watch TV, or to listen to music. He walked to meals alone and wouldn’t speak to anyone. The nurse prescribed antidepressants for him, but he would not take them.

He was having car accidents, but the family couldn’t talk him into giving up his car keys.

One evening Marie turned on the local news to see her father in an upside-down car, hanging from his seat belt. He was interviewed by the newsman on site, but denied being hurt. He never mentioned it to any of them. Finally, after one more accident, the Oklahoma highway patrolman who investigated it explained the possible consequences to him in words he could understand and he subsequently gave his car to Nancy.

A few months later, Nancy told Marie that their father had stopped paying rent and his electric bill at the assisted living apartment he lived in. Nancy received a call from the manager, and went there to see what she could do. She had been visiting him often and he came to her house for meals and visits, but this came out of left field. She had no idea he had not been paying his bills.

"Daddy," she said, "why don't you give me a power of attorney so I can help you pay your bills?"

He blew up at that. "You already got my car, and now you are trying to steal my money!"

She told Marie he was yelling at her right in the reception area. Nancy just left it alone after that, figuring it would somehow work out. A week later, Nancy got a phone call from the hospital, and called Marie and the other siblings.

"Daddy's in the hospital, and they say he isn't too sick. He is in for observation. I went up there to see him and the nurses and nurses' aides were all telling me how nice and how pleasant he is, and I told them that if that were the case, he was dying. They didn't believe me, but I thought you all should know."

Two days later, Nancy called Marie. "You know what I told you? Daddy died a few hours ago."

"What happened?" Marie said.

"They aren't real sure. It will have to wait for an autopsy. I will call the others and start to make plans for the funeral, if that is all right will you all."

"Yes, thanks for calling and for taking that on. I appreciate it. Let me know about the funeral."

After Marie hung up, she realized that it was exactly 51 weeks since her mother died. He was not going to face the anniversary of her death.

Chapter Forty-Three

The grown-up children gathered to bury their father, to dispose of his belongings and to give Tim, the executor, a chance to consult with them about the will. Nancy, who lived in the town where he died, handled most of it. They agreed it was tragic he had lived such an unhappy life.

After perusing the will, Tim gathered them together and said, "Daddy left four CDs, one each for Ann, me, Marie, and Shirley. Nothing for Nancy." When Tim told them that, there was a dead silence. No one knew what to say. Finally, Tim said, "Why don't we put the money together and divide it five ways, with a share going to Nancy?" Everyone was relieved and agreed that was the best solution.

Nancy, a single mother of two girls, when she could breathe again, thanked them all.

When it was all worked out, Marie's share was a little over twenty-five thousand dollars. She knew exactly what she was going to do with the money. She always wanted a house and this was the best chance she would ever have to buy one.

She started looked in the newspaper the weekend after the funeral. To her surprise, she found one that sounded perfect, close to her job. MedPrime recently completed a new building, with up-to-date studio facilities and plenty of room for all its employees. Marie had her own cubicle, and the writers were segregated from the producers so they could concentrate.

Ruth surprised everyone when she announced: "Guess what? I'm getting married!"

"Great news!" said Marie.

Her bosses were happy to see her go and joined in the chorus of congratulations. Everyone was completely astonished because she never mentioned dating anyone special. She gave a month's notice and started training Marie in the aspects of the job that Ruth had always handled.

Meanwhile, Charlotte told Ruth, "I've found another job and will also be leaving in two weeks."

Marie felt like the floor was falling out from under her. She had a lot to learn and a lot to do. Marie really didn't have time to find another employee, but she knew the receptionist, Flo, at MedPrime was a PhD candidate in English at Oklahoma City University.

She asked Caroline, "How would it be if I offered the job to Florence?"

Caroline said, "Is she qualified?"

"Flo has a degree in English and is working on her PhD. In fact, she has done everything but her dissertation. I know this job would pay more than her receptionist gig."

"Sure, go ahead, it will save us a lot of trouble."

Without even waiting for Florence's break, Marie went straight to the front desk and said, "Flo, we have an opening in our writer's unit, and I want to offer it to you first. It will be a big pay raise for you and allow you to use your degree."

To her consternation, Flo didn't seem excited about the opportunity. In fact, she was reluctant to talk about the job. "I am happy in this receptionist job; I have done it for two years and I'm not sure I want to change."

"Flo, think about the money and that you would be writing for a living. It's got to be more interesting than this." Marie swept her hands open to indicate the large desk and telephones Flo was presiding over now.

"Okay, I'll think about it and talk to my family tonight. I'll let you know Monday."

"Thanks, Flo."

Caroline was also surprised to learn that not only was Flo not instantly interested in the job, but they decided to wait before they advertised the it.

On Saturday, Marie contacted the realtor who held the listing for the house she was interested in. When she looked at it, she fell completely in love with it; a three-bedroom, two bath, small house with a big living room and a dining room with one glass outside wall. The backyard was surrounded by hedges, so it was remote from the neighbors. It would be a perfect place to entertain Mensans.

It needed a lot of work. She called Shirley, whose talent was decorating, and she came over as soon as she could, even though it was in a driving rainstorm. Marie walked her around the house, describing it to her, and then took her to the glass wall so she could see the dining room, living room, and the kitchen.

"Oh, this is a darling place! We can do all kinds of things with it. You should definitely buy it if you want it. It needs new carpet and new paint and some wallpaper, but I can help you with all of that."

Marie started the process of buying the home with the inspection, finding a realtor of her own and applying for a bank loan. She was a little lost, since it was the first time she had bought a house, but she was determined not to let this one get away. It had been so neglected, the price was only in the eighty thousands, and she knew she wouldn't find another like it only a mile from her job.

Back at work, Flo came to Marie and said, "Well, I talked it over with my son and decided to take the job."

"Oh, that's great, Flo. Let me know how soon you can start work. I'll tell Caroline."

Marie learned as much as she could as fast as she could from Ruth. As soon as Ruth and Charlotte were gone, Flo came to work with her. While Marie was working to make the deadlines and get everything done correctly, she had to teach Flo her job. Luckily, Flo caught on quickly and was able to do some of the work right away.

About a month later, at Christmas, Marie just barely got the packets of syllabi to the printers. She had taken off a full week so she could move. One of the things she wanted to do was to paint before she got her furniture into the new house.

Flo asked Caroline, “Now that there isn’t a lot to do, could I work on my dissertation during the down days between Christmas and New Year’s?”

“Sure,” Caroline answered, “as long as you are here every day to take care of anything that comes up.”

When Marie took off, she cajoled Shirley into spending her vacation painting. She painted every room a different color, and while she painted the bathrooms, Shirley made curtains for the windows and put up wallpaper borders. When they finished, the house was completely changed. She needed new carpeting, but the rest of the house was lovely. Shirley could work miracles with just a little money.

Marie now had a kitchen, two bedrooms, a study, a dining room, and a large living room. Outside, a fence delineated her small backyard. At the rear, Marie planted morning glories, which bloomed all summer and into the fall. She had a sprinkler system in the front yard. The wooden fence enclosed the yard, and became wrought iron as it passed her front door, with a locked gate in front of her porch. It made her feel safe and meant that no one could approach the front door without her knowing about it.

The front yard was an expanse of grass, while the back yard was filled with tall bushes and trailing multi-colored flowers. Outside the windows alongside the living and dining room, there was a patio. It was a wonderful house for entertaining.

Marie was so happy in it, even when she was just working on her computer in the study with the soft green walls.

Around New Year's, Marie moved. As soon as the movers got her things into the house, the phone rang. It was a clerk at the job, asking a question. "Ask Flo. She should be able to help you."

"I don't know where Flo is; we haven't seen her."

"Then just use your best judgment."

Marie wondered about Flo not being around, but she had a ton of stuff to do, so she just put it out of her mind. While she was unpacking on New Year's Eve, the clerk called her back. "The printer is here. He needs some help with the packet."

"Get Flo to help him."

"I don't know where Flo is."

"Okay, tell him I will be there in twenty minutes."

The printers had left their newest guy alone over the holidays to get out the packet, and he needed advice on how to do it. Marie worked with him about four hours, when they finally got it straightened out. There was no sign of Flo anywhere.

Marie spent that night and the next day unpacking, and finally had things squared away just as it was time to return to work. When she got in, Flo was seated at her desk. "Where have you been?"

"You know Caroline gave me permission to work on my dissertation."

"Caroline gave you permission to work on it here, not at home. You were supposed to be here in case anything came up. I suppose you knew Caroline was taking the whole two weeks off."

"I knew nothing would happen so I just stayed at home and worked," Flo said.

"Well, something did happen and I had to come up here and work in the middle of my move."

"Oh, I'm sorry."

"Generally, I would tell Caroline, but I know how angry it would make her and I'm afraid she would fire you. Since I don't want that to happen I won't tell her what you did. But don't ever do anything like that again."

Marie would never completely trust her again.

Chapter Forty-Four

Marie bought new carpet and found furniture at a used furniture store that sold hotel furniture, she got some lovely desks and nice little green loveseat and chair for the study, and a durable cherry bedroom suite that matched the bed Tim gave her, and a couple of sofas and chairs for the living room.

She started having a Mensa gathering of some sort about once a month. Her living room was large, with a sixteen-foot ceiling, and having two bathrooms made it a convenient gathering place. There was plenty of room for people to spread out. Marie enjoyed hosting parties after all these years of going to others' houses and not reciprocating.

At one party, she noticed a good-looking, quiet guy sitting in a corner by himself in her living room. He was tall, with short blond hair and wore glasses. Marie went over to him,

"Hi, I'm the hostess, Marie."

"I'm Brad, and I'm new to the group. Just moved here."

As hostess, though, she didn't have much time to spend with him that night, but she watched him covertly because she was interested in getting to know him.

At work, Marie put in long hours; training Flo and making sure everything was the deadline were met. Flo was some help, but most of the work fell to her. Some things just didn't get done, but the syllabi were done on time each month.

On the weekends, she still had time to get to Mensa functions. On a Sunday night at an event, she ran into Brad. He said, “You know, I really enjoy the stories you write for the newsletter. They are really good.”

“Why thank you, Brad, that is really nice. I wrote one about the Supreme Court I was thinking about using, but not the latest decisions they have made.”

“ Whoa, wait a minute, I like those decisions.” Then they got into a political discussion. They weren’t finished talking when the meeting was over, so he asked her to go out to a coffeehouse with him. They continued their conversation, and he bought her strawberries in cream. They weren’t quite on the same page politically, but he was making the right moves otherwise.

After they talked for a couple of hours, both of them telling each other about their lives,

Brad asked, “Would you go out with me if I asked you for a date?”

“Yes, I would, but…” Marie didn’t want to start anything with Brad unless he knew of her bipolar disorder. He was so attractive she didn’t want him to leave as soon as he found out. Might as well get it over with.

“Brad, you should know I have bipolar disorder. I was diagnosed several years ago and am taking medication. I am doing well and have been stable for years.’

Instead of the usual questions, Brad said, “That is no problem for me. As a matter of fact, my roommate, Stan, is bipolar. I understand a lot of the problems that go along with it. That wouldn’t bother me.”

“I didn’t know you had a roommate.”

“Yes, he is a friend of mine who does better when he lives with someone. He is a teacher; sometimes he has to walk half the night. I understand when he is a little manic. I also have a sixteen-year old son, Ben, who spends alternate weekends with me. I want you to meet both of them.”

"I would be happy to, but now you better take me back to my car. Tomorrow's a work day."

"Okay, but how about going out to dinner with me next Saturday? At six o'clock?"

"I'd love to. How should I dress?"

"Casually—we aren't going anyplace too fancy."

Marie enjoyed her time with Brad. Even though he was in charge of IT at Xerox, he didn't talk down to her as so many others in that field did. He made a point of telling her he enjoyed her stories and seemed interested in talking with her. She looked forward to their date that weekend.

After several months of success with Flo working on the syllabi, Marie was surprised at a staff meeting.

Caroline called her out and gave her a light blue plastic award paperweight for her desk etched with "Marie—Dependable, Dedicated, & Determined." She was named "lead writer," and was given two dinners at Ruth Criss' Steakhouse. After this happened, Caroline said, "Come to my office after the meeting."

Marie went to Caroline's office, curious as to what she was wanted for after all that. She was happy; this one meeting made up for all the years she had trouble holding a job. When she got there, Caroline said, "I have news for you. I put in for a raise for you when I saw how well you handled things. You have done a great job and I think you should be rewarded. You will get your raise in two weeks. It will be ten thousand dollars a year."

Marie gasped, "Thank you, thank you. I don't know what else to say. This has really been a day. I appreciate it—all of it—so much. Caroline, this is such a surprise."

"I just want you to know that I realize how hard you have worked and we want to keep you around. Now go and enjoy your dinner."

"Again, thank you, Caroline."

Marie had to take a vacation or lose the time, so she grabbed résumés off Monster.com and hired another writer, Nate, who could start work right away. There was little time to train him and after the deadlines, she would go on her one-week vacation, Flo would continue working with him.

That same week they were treated to an unusual heat wave. Saturday had a high of one hundred and fifteen degrees. Marie's air conditioner could only cool to eighty-five degrees, but she was grateful that it was working at all.

Marie was nervous about her first date with Brad. Ready early, she went to the front of the house to peek out the window. It was seven minutes to six when he pulled up in his light green Camry. She expected him to come to the door, but soon it became obvious that he was going to wait until straight up six o'clock. So he sat in the car, in that heat, until it was time for him to pick her up.

Marie admired his manners, but wouldn't have minded at all if he had made a run for the air-conditioning. They went to an Italian restaurant, but neither anticipated that the entire city was at restaurants that evening instead of heating up their kitchens so they had to wait quite a while to be served. But it was cool while they waited.

They talked about their lives while they waited and while they ate, how much they had in common, and that they liked each other. After dinner, he came in and played with the cats, laughing when Peave got cat hair all over his shirt.

"When can I see you again?"

"I am going on vacation, so tomorrow I have to pack. My sister, Shirley, works at a company that has a special arrangement with the Hilton in Galveston. She reserved our rooms at a discount right on the seawall."

"That sounds like a good deal. When will you be back?'

"Thursday, in the afternoon."

"Can I call you then?"

"Sure, I'd love to hear from you."

They hugged goodbye, and Marie was a little sorry about the timing of her vacation.

The next morning, Marie and Shirley began the long drive to Galveston, It was one of their favorite places, and even more attractive because of the discounts. When they were children, they went to Galveston every year because their mother came from Houston and one of the conditions of marrying Marie's father and living in Oklahoma City was that she visit her beloved Gulf yearly.

When they finally got there, Galveston was having the hottest day they had ever had, breaking all records, but it was several degrees cooler than it was at home, and the sea breeze was blowing. It seemed a lot cooler to Marie and Shirley.

"What a nice cool breeze you have here," Shirley commented. The clerk rolled her eyes.

All the four days they were in Galveston, they got up at dawn and went for an early morning walk on the beach. They ate breakfast at a little place they found, went swimming and playing in the water until midday, when they took a nap. Then it was lunchtime. In the evening, back to the beach, just as when they were children, they couldn't get enough of the beach and the salty air and water.

When it was time to leave, they were glad to be getting home and back to their cats. Marie was feeling rested, but would have loved a little more time off work. She wondered on the drive home if she would hear from Brad.

The cats were glad to have her back so Marie spent some time petting them. She washed her sandy clothes, while listening for the phone.

At about six, Brad called. "How was your vacation?"

"It was great; I have to go back to work tomorrow."

"That's always the worst part. Listen, I don't have Ben, my son, next weekend, so let's go out tomorrow night."

"Okay."

"We'll take in a movie, and then get something to eat. I'll pick you up at six again."

"I'll see you then."

With her spirits lifted, Marie continued to get ready for work the next day. When she got into the office the next morning, she greeted everyone and told them about her vacation. Then the receptionist called her. "Come down here, there is something here for you."

"What is it?"

"Just come here. You'll see."

Marie went to the front desk and was surprised when the receptionist handed her a flower arrangement. It was from Brad. Marie had never been courted like this before, and he was getting to her.

When he picked her up Friday night, he had more flowers in his hands. "Oh, thank you. How pretty!"

Marie completely surprised. They had a good time on their date, and this time he stayed over. Marie told herself it would be a good idea to move things around in the garage so he could park his car there in the future. The next morning, he took her out for breakfast, to a special Mexican restaurant that made killer breakfast burritos.

It was too late for Marie to make up her mind, she was already in love. He was so caring and accepting that he would be able to handle anything. She thought to herself, I could tell this guy I had breast cancer and it wouldn't scare him off. Marie relaxed into the relationship.

Chapter Forty-Five

While Marie loved her job, things did not always go smoothly at work. In that respect, it was like any other position. When new material came to Marie through the mail or email, she would ask who could format it. In the majority of cases, both Nate and Flo said, "I'm already working on something," or, "I'm too busy." Marie would take it on herself. She did about fifty percent of the work, instead of thirty percent.

Lousy at proofing what she wrote, Marie threw extra proofing on the others. They did it, but there were resentments all around. They also had a tendency to get short with one another around deadlines. However, generally, they pulled together to make certain that everything was done correctly and on time.

Sometimes it was hard to please the customers, although most were happy with the writing. Some of them, usually the ones who sent the least information, were picky about the format of their syllabus. The company just went with the premise that the customer was always right. For example, it took a sharp eye to discern that the presenter used the word "discreet" when he meant "discrete" and to make that correction without hurting anyone's feelings. It was all part of the job.

Marie and Brad's relationship continued to grow and at Christmastime, he surprised her with a trip to the Atlantis resort in Nassau. "Pack for warm weather and bring a bathing suit." That's all he told her and she didn't know where they were going until they boarded the plane.

At the resort, she was enchanted by the glass aquarium tunnel a person could walk through, surrounded on all sides by colorful tropical fish and could have watched them for hours. Brad was amused by her childlike delight in the water slides that went down the sides of the building and dumped her into the clear blue water. Marie loved the beaches and he could only get her inside to rest, eat and sleep. Her mother had taught her to eat only fresh seafood, and she loved the variety of it. They watched the gorgeous sunsets in the evenings and had slow, easy sex in the afternoons when it was lazy and hot outside. They weren't nearly ready to go when it was time to go home.

"Brad. I can't thank you enough for that trip," Marie said, hugging him as they packed to go back to the City. "I have never enjoyed a vacation more."

"Don't you think I enjoyed it too? It was a lot of fun for me. I brought Ben down here last year and we had a ball. I knew you would like it."

They went back to regular life, which included a lot of Mensa activities. Marie had been appointed to the "New Members' Chair," which meant she contacted each new member by mail with a welcome letter and information about Mensa. Her position also called for her to host two New Members' parties a year; parties which attracted over a hundred persons apiece and served a ton of food and beer.

Brad had been elected to the Board, and that took up a lot of his time. They went to Mensa parties or events every weekend, sometimes taking Ben along with them. He enjoyed meeting some of the teenage Mensans, and planned to take the test so he could join.

One weekend Marie noticed that her car had that hesitation in starting that usually means the battery is low. She knew her battery was years old, so she asked, "Brad, will you go with me to help me pick out a good-enough battery? I'm not too good at maintaining cars, I just know the basics."

Brad went with her, but instead of helping her make a decision, he said to the service man, "Just install the top-of-the-line battery, and I'll pay for it."

"No," Marie said, "that is not why I asked for your help. I just wanted your advice."

Brad brushed her off. "I'm happy to help you with your car whenever you need it."

That made her feel even more secure, because one of her biggest fears was dealing with car problems. Marie was always afraid she would be taken advantage of due to her lack of knowledge.

Brad and Marie had their first fight over a story she wrote for the local newsletter. He said he enjoyed her stories and encouraged her writing, but this time he was angry. "Why did you write about your old boyfriend this month? Everyone in the group but me knows him. It makes me look stupid."

"No, Brad, it was supposed to be a funny story about the time my car broke down in Paul's Valley and Matt offered to fly up and take me home, and I got all insulted that he thought I couldn't handle a car-breakdown problem and told him I would manage it myself. I had to give in after all and have him come rescue me."

"Well, I don't have a plane so I guess I couldn't have helped you."

"Brad, I certainly wouldn't have written it if I had known that it would upset you. I was only trying to be funny."

"It wasn't funny to me."

Then he stalked off. Marie thought it silly of him to blame her for writing a story that mentioned a guy she used to date. By now, the guy had moved to Washington, D.C. and she hadn't seen him in years. Brad felt it was rude of her to mention her old boyfriend to a group of all their mutual friends, leaving him at a disadvantage when he didn't even know the man.

They didn't speak to each other for two days. Finally Marie, thinking it was too dumb, called him at work, "Brad, this is ridiculous, we are both being stupid. Isn't our relationship more important than a story I wrote that was half-fiction anyway?"

"Yeah, I guess I got my feeling hurt. It is pretty dumb. I'll come over after work and we can talk about it."

When Brad arrived, there wasn't any talking. They moved into each other's arms and the making up made the fight worthwhile.

Oklahoma City was doing a great deal of restoration work downtown. In the warehouse district, city leaders hoped to attract hotels, restaurants, and retailers to fill the mostly empty buildings. To start, they were dredging a canal through the area, which they thought would help in attracting foot traffic. It would add beauty to the area and make it seem cooler in the summer.

Saturday night, Brad suggested that they have dinner at the one restaurant that had moved into that area at that time, the "Spaghetti Warehouse." "We both love the food, and we can check out the progress of the work they are doing."

"That sounds like fun."

At the restaurant, Marie had her favorite, spaghetti and meatballs, and Brad had pasta carbonera. They didn't talk much, just enjoyed the food and each other's company. Their relationship had progressed to the point that they could just be quiet with one another; they didn't have to talk to each other all the time. Finally, they finished and Brad said, "Why don't we walk over to the canal and see what they have done?"

"I'd like that."

They strolled over to the canal, and found the dredging was finished. All around it there were all kinds of new plants and foliage and spindly little trees. There were elm and oak and redbud and sycamore. It looked raw and incomplete, but Marie exclaimed, “Oh, in a few years, this will be all shady and beautiful!”

“Then will you come back and see it with me?”

Marie turned to answer. Puzzled, she saw Brad down on one knee. He held a ring, then took her hand and slipped it on her finger.

This time Marie didn’t say “no.”

The End

www.ingramcontent.com/pod-product-compliance
Lightning Source LLC
Chambersburg PA
CBHW051446170526
45166CB00001B/129

* 9 7 8 1 4 7 7 6 6 1 5 6 7 *